Surgery of the Rheumatoid Hand and Wrist

Surgery of the Rheumatoid Hand and Wrist

Course papers presented at the XIth Congress of the Federation of the European Societies for Surgery of the Hand

FESSH Instructional Course Book

Editors:

Ian Trail
Wrightington Hospital
Hall Lane
Appley Bridge
Wigan WN6 9EP
UNITED KINGDOM

Michael Hayton
Wrightington Hospital
Hall Lane
Appley Bridge
Wigan WN6 9EP
UNITED KINGDOM

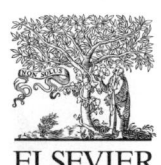

ELSEVIER

2006

ELSEVIER B.V.
Radarweg 29
P.O. Box 211, 1000 AE Amsterdam
The Netherlands

ELSEVIER Inc.
525 B Street, Suite 1900
San Diego, CA 92101-4495
USA

ELSEVIER Ltd
The Boulevard, Langford Lane
Kidlington, Oxford OX5 1GB
UK

ELSEVIER Ltd
84 Theobalds Road
London WC1X 8RR
UK

First edition 2006

Library of Congress Cataloging in Publication Data
A catalog record from the Library of Congress has been applied for.

British Library Cataloguing in Publication Data
A catalogue record from the British Library has been applied for.

International Congress Series No. 1295
ISBN: 0-444-52852-0/978-0-444-52852-0
ISSN: 0531-5131

⊗ The paper used in this publication meets the requirements of ANSI/NISO Z39.48-1992 (Permanence of Paper).
Printed in The Netherlands.

Contents

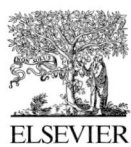

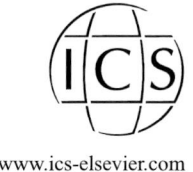

www.ics-elsevier.com

Preface

Inflammatory arthritis continues to inflict a serious burden of disability on many patients. Recent advances in medical therapy are beginning to alter the pattern of the disease presented to hand surgeons, but the need for effective reconstructive hand and wrist surgery continues. Inflammatory arthritis produces challenging problems in the hand and wrist for the patient's daily activities, and also for the surgeon who advises on treatment. Maintaining satisfactory hand function tests the skills and knowledge of the surgeon in both decision-making and surgical technique.

The chapters in this book are written by the faculty at the Instructional Course of the FESSH Congress in 2006. This international group of experts has distilled the current status of diagnosis and treatment of inflammatory arthritis as it affects the hand and wrist. Professor Roger Sturrock covers the current status of diagnosis and medical therapy for inflammatory arthritis. Several of the surgical authors are leaders in the development of new replacement arthroplasties and are well placed to describe the benefits and risks. The emphasis on indications, surgical techniques, results and complications will be of particular interest to surgeons who treat inflammatory arthritis. Other chapters deal with the management of the more classic problems of the rheumatoid hand, especially tendon and soft-tissue abnormalities, and also cover the role of rehabilitation.

We hope that these contributions will help clinicians caring for the many patients suffering from inflammatory arthritis, encourage close collaboration between rheumatologist and surgeon, and stimulate further investigation and improvement in our treatments.

Ian Trail
Editor

0531-5131/ © 2006 Published by Elsevier B.V.
doi:10.1016/j.ics.2006.05.002

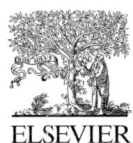

International Congress Series 1295 (2006) 1–8

ELSEVIER

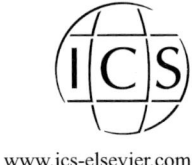

www.ics-elsevier.com

Update on the pathogenesis of rheumatoid arthritis

Roger D. Sturrock

University of Glasgow, UK

Abstract. Inflammatory joint diseases are complex, but considerable advances have been made in the understanding of the pathophysiology of diseases such as rheumatoid arthritis. This has led to considerable improvements in therapy and an improvement in long-term outcome for patients with inflammatory joint disease. Other rheumatic diseases such as psoriatic arthritis, ankylosing spondylitis and juvenile idiopathic arthritis have also been the subject of advances in therapy. © 2006 Elsevier B.V. All rights reserved.

Keywords: Inflammatory joint disease; Immunopathology; Biologic therapy

1. Introduction

The aetiology of rheumatoid arthritis (RA) is unknown, but much is now understood regarding its immunopathology.

The disease is an outcome of the inter-relationship between genetics, environment (? infectious trigger) and dysregulation of the immune system (Fig. 1).

An inflammatory synovitis is the hallmark of RA and, in the early phase of the disease, the synovium is infiltrated by lymphocytes, macrophages and polymorphonuclear cells (PMNs) as well as increased expression of cytokines such as TNFα (Fig. 2).

As the disease becomes established, cartilage and bone erosion occur associated with a proliferative synovitis and the release of proteolytic enzymes. An excess of synovial fluid production is a feature of active RA and there is an imbalance between the production of pro- and anti-inflammatory cytokines with the balance being shifted in favour of the pro-inflammatory cytokines such as IL-1, IL-6 and TNFα (Fig. 3).

There is a dysregulation of the T-cell network with activation of TH1 cells and also proliferation of B cells and fibroblasts with the production of auto-antibodies such as rheumatoid factors (RF). New blood vessel formation occurs as part of the inflammatory

---

E-mail address: r.d.sturrock@clinmed.gla.ac.uk.

0531-5131/ © 2006 Elsevier B.V. All rights reserved.
doi:10.1016/j.ics.2006.03.070

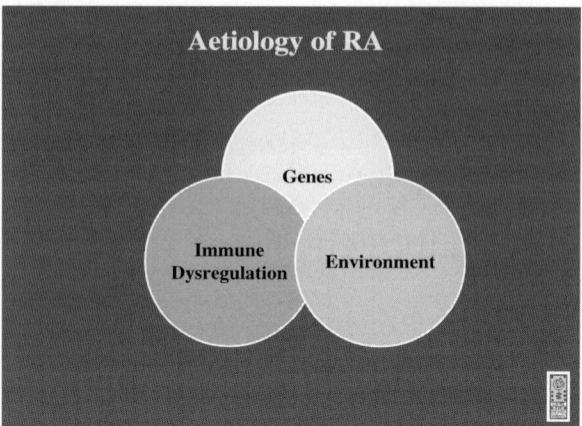

Fig. 1.

pannus that invades the articular cartilage. The upregulation of adhesion molecules on the endothelium leads to the ingress of PMNs from the peripheral circulation in to the synovial cavity (Fig. 4).

Extra-articular features such as anaemia, weight loss and sometimes low grade fever are results of the acute phase response driven by the pro-inflammatory cytokines, while vasculitis is a result of complement activation and immune complex deposition.

1.1. Genetics

The class II HLA antigens DRB1*0404 and DRB1*0401 are strongly linked to RA and are expressed on dendritic cells that have the key role of presenting antigen to TH1 cells with their consequent activation. The HLA DR-B1 alleles share a common amino acid sequence at positions 70–74, which is known as the shared epitope (SE) and is associated with severe destructive RA. Patients with either of these two HLA antigens are more likely

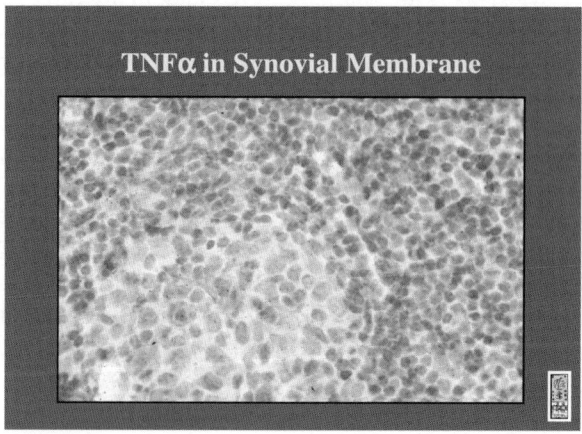

Fig. 2.

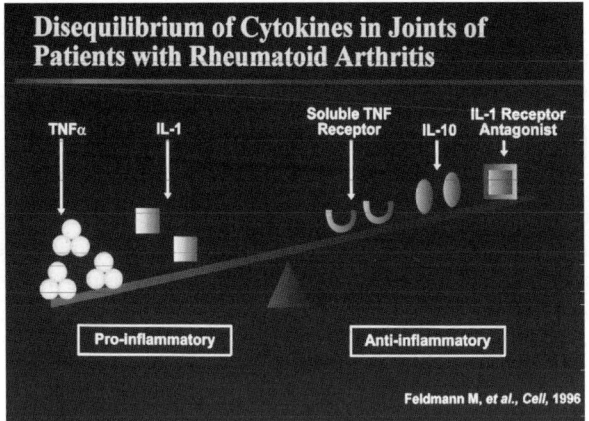

Fig. 3.

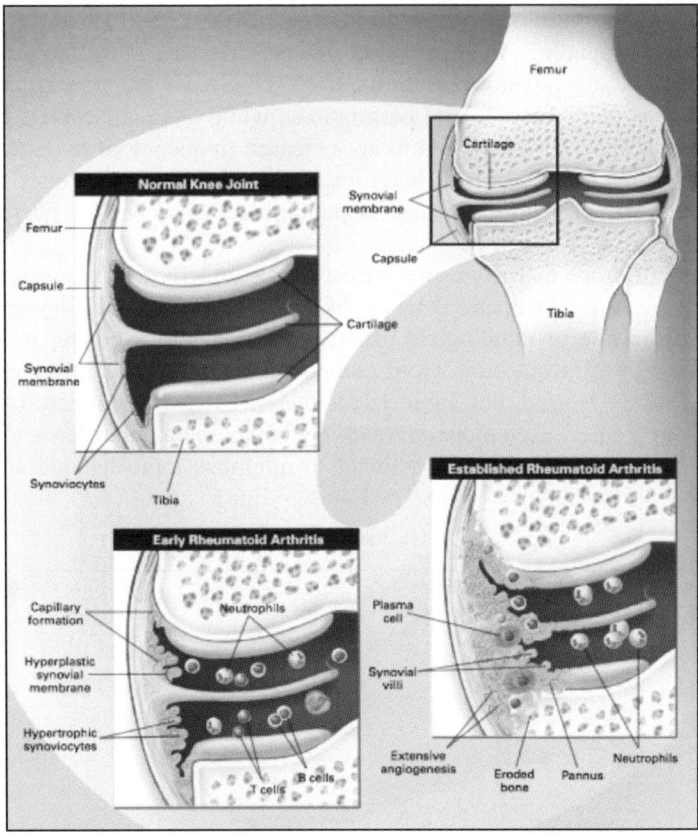

Fig. 4. (Taken from Choy and Panayi in Mechanisms of Disease, NEJM, 2001, 344, 12.)

to have severe RA and to be seropositive for RF and other antibodies such as to citrullinated proteins (anti-ccp). Anti-CCP antibodies may develop very early in the disease process prior to the expression of RF and are increasingly being used as a sensitive and specific test for RA patients with synovitis of less than 6-month duration.

1.2. Co-morbidity

RA is a systemic disease, and pulmonary, cardiovascular and neurological complications may occur in severe disease. A normochromic, normocytic anaemia is inversely related to a persistently elevated ESR and CRP. It has recently become apparent that cardiovascular complications such as hypertension, myocardial infarction and stroke are increased in frequency in RA and associated with the chronic acute phase response seen in continuing disease.

2. Current medical therapy

The aim of drug therapy for RA is to relieve the symptoms of pain, stiffness and joint swelling, and to prevent cartilage damage and bone erosion occurring within the joints. Non-steroidal anti-inflammatory drugs (NSAIDs) are used as symptom relievers, but they do not have any effect on disease progression. The NSAIDs are divided into COX-1 and COX-2 inhibitors depending on their mode of action on the enzyme cyclooxygenase, which is involved in prostaglandin synthesis. COX-1 NSAIDs are associated with gastric side effects such as ulcers, bleeds and perforations, while COX-2 NSAIDs have a lower gastric toxicity but appear to be linked to an increased frequency of hypertension, stroke and myocardial infarction. NSAIDs therefore have to be used cautiously and avoided where possible in patients with a history of peptic ulcer or ischaemic heart disease and hypertension.

Another class of drugs that have some effect on the underlying disease process are the Disease Modifying Anti-Rheumatic Drugs (DMARDs). These have a slow onset of action and slow down the rate of radiological progression of RA to a greater or lesser extent depending on the drug in question. Gold compounds and subsequently D-penicillamine were the first DMARDs used, but Table 1 lists the DMARDs in standard use:

The DMARDs are now used more aggressively in the treatment of RA and are initiated early on in the disease process in an attempt to minimise joint damage and functional

Table 1

Commonly used DMARDs
Hydroxychloroquine
Sulphasalazine
Methotrexate
Less commonly used
Gold
D-Penicillamine
Azathioprine
Cyclosporin
Minocycline
Leflunomide

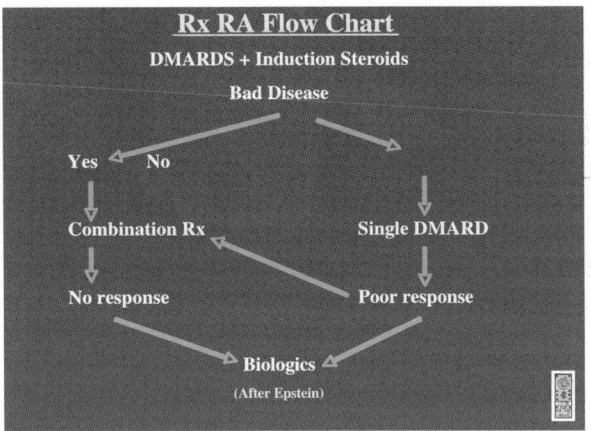

Fig. 5.

incapacity. Side effects include neutropenia and thrombocytopenia, and they require careful monitoring. They are frequently used in combination often with steroids in the first 3 months of therapy. A modern treatment paradigm for RA is illustrated in Fig. 5.

In the last 10 years, a new series of compounds specifically targeted at the pro-inflammatory cytokines TNFα and IL-1 have been developed and used in the treatment of RA. These are known as the biologic agents, and the three anti-TNF blocking drugs in common use are Infliximab, Etanercept and Adalumimab. They are either given by intravenous infusion or by subcutaneous injection (Table 2).

These biologic agents are given in combination with Methotrexate, and have been shown to significantly slow down the progression of joint damage, improve functional capacity and decrease fatigue levels in RA patients. However, there is a slightly increased risk of infection particularly tuberculosis and so patients suitable for these therapies require to be screened for past or present TB.

Other biologic agents are in phase 2 and 3 trials and include drugs targeted at IL-6 and adhesion molecules. A monoclonal antibody directed against B cells (Rituximab) is also an effective agent in the treatment of severe RA resistant to TNF blockade.

3. Implications for joint surgery

The early use of DMARDs and the biologic agents has reduced the need for synovectomy and there is some anecdotal evidence that the need for major joint replacement therapy has declined in younger patients who have been treated aggressively. However, there is a large cohort of patients with secondary osteoarthritis who require

Table 2

Drug	Route	Dosage
Infliximab	i.v.	3 mg/kg every 8 weeks
Etanercept	s.c.	25 mg twice a week
Adalumimab	s.c.	40 mg every 2 weeks

surgical intervention. The continued use of DMARDs during surgery does not increase the risk of infection but the biologic agents should be stopped temporarily over the period of surgery—ideally 2–3 weeks prior to surgery and recommenced once wound healing has taken place. Patients on steroid therapy will require an increase in their dosage in the perioperative period.

4. Other inflammatory arthropathies

The three conditions that may create a surgical demand are:

1. Psoriatic arthritis
2. Ankylosing spondylitis
3. Juvenile idiopathic arthritis (formerly known as Still's disease).

5. Psoriatic arthritis

Brief notes on this inflammatory arthopathy:

- Arthritis occurs in approximately 15% of patients with psoriasis.
- Seronegative disease.
- Usually an oligoarthritis with an asymmetrical presentation.
- Associated with psoriatic nail changes (Fig. 6).
- In the hands and feet, there is distal interphalyngeal (DIP) joint involvement.
- Spinal inflammatory disease similar to ankylosing spondylitis can occur.
- There is a severe destructive form of the disease—arthritis mutilans.
- Treatment is with DMARDs such as Methotrexate and Sulphasalazine. Anti-TNF therapy can be very effective as an adjunct.

6. Ankylosing spondylitis

Brief notes:

- Predominantly a disease of young men, male/female 3:1.
- Strong genetic component—95% patients are HLA B27 positive.

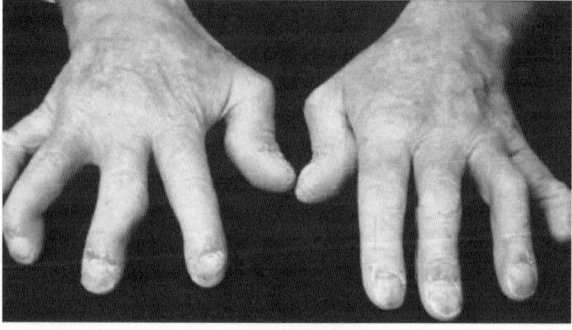

Fig. 6.

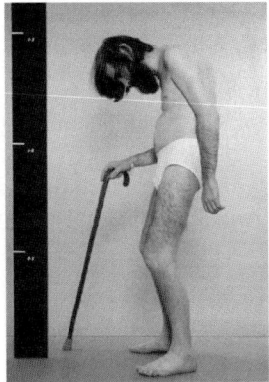

Fig. 7.

- Inflammatory back pain.
- Characteristic posture in severe disease (Fig. 7).
- MRI scan shows early sacroiliitis with inflammation before pelvic X-rays become abnormal.
- 20% have hip disease.
- Treatment is with physio and NSAIDs.
- Severe cases respond well to anti-TNF therapy.

7. Juvenile idiopathic arthritis (JIA)

Brief notes:

- Several forms of the disease:
    Systemic
    Pauciarticular
    Extended pauciarticular

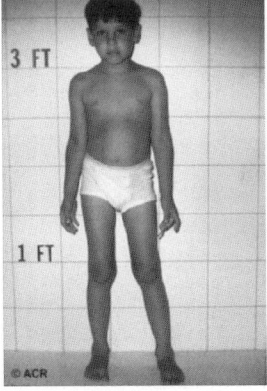

Fig. 8.

Polyarticular

Enthesis-related arthritis

- Occurs in children under the age of 16.
- May affect growth and development of limbs and digits (Fig. 8).
- Can persist into adult life.
- Some patients develop rapid cartilage loss in hips and knees.
- Treatment is with DMARDs. Anti-TNF therapy now widely used with good effect.

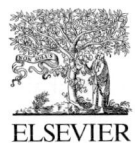

International Congress Series 1295 (2006) 9–26

ELSEVIER

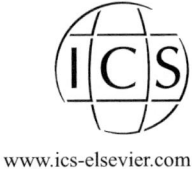

www.ics-elsevier.com

Examination of the rheumatoid hand and wrist

Alberto Lluch *

Institut Kaplan, Paseo Bonanova, 9, 08022 Barcelona, Spain

Abstract. Rheumatoid disease affects almost all of the musculoskeletal system as well as some internal organs, such as the heart and lungs, pleura, eyes, lymph nodes and vessels. In the case of the upper extremity, we should know the time of onset and type of disease, as the extent and degree of tissue involvement varies among the different types of rheumatoid disease. Surgical treatment and postoperative management will vary significantly in patients suffering from sclerodermia to those of systemic lupus erythematosus. This can also be said about the type of medication used for treating the disease, as more recent medications may alter collagen synthesis and infection rates. Before examining the hand, shoulder and elbow function should also be assessed. Clinical examination of the hand joints is most important, as all deformities, including most tendon ruptures and tendon dislocations are secondary to joint involvement. We should carefully examine for the presence and intensity of joint synovitis, and the degree of joint deformity and record the range of active and passive joint mobility. Radiological examination should be done in all cases to determine the degree of joint cartilage destruction, joint subluxation, and even joint ankylosis which is some times difficult to asses on clinical examination due to a fixed joint deformity from extraarticular causes. CAT scan examination can be useful for wrist joint assessment. Magnetic resonance examinations may be required only in certain circumstances, i.e. to determine the presence of joint or tendon synovitis not clearly assessed by clinical exploration, and the location of a flexor tendon rupture. © 2006 Elsevier B.V. All rights reserved.

Keywords: Rheumatoid hand; Rheumatoid wrist; Clinical examination

1. Clinical examination

1.1. Skin examination

First the skin should be examined, to determine its thickness and texture, presence of ecchymosis or petechial hemorrhages, rheumatoid nodules, vasculitis, Raynaud's

---

* Tel.: +34 93 417 84 84; fax: +34 93 211 04 02.
  E-mail addresses: albertolluch@infonegocio.com, alluch@telefonica.net.

phenomenon, etc. The presence and extent of psoriatic lesions, in both skin and nails should also be recorded.

1.2. Nerve examination

Possible sites of nerve compression are found at the ulnar nerve in the elbow, the median nerve at the wrist and the radial nerve at the proximal forearm, underneath the aponeurotic origin of the supinator muscle, known as the arcade of Frohse. The clinical manifestations of sensory nerve compressions are pain, paraesthesia, hyposthesia and anesthesia. Clinical manifestations of motor nerve compressions are pain, muscle weakness, muscle paralysis and muscle atrophy depending on the degree and duration of the compression.

Compression of the median nerve, carrying both sensory and motor fibers, can be experienced at the onset of the disease, but it becomes rare at later stages, due to the fact that the hypertrophic synovium around the finger flexor tendons will attenuate the flexor retinaculum, thus enlarging the dimension of the carpal tunnel and releasing nerve compression.

Compression of the ulnar nerve at the elbow, carrying both sensory and motor fibers, is also rare, even in cases of severe elbow joint involvement, due to similar anatomical changes caused by the underlying joint synovitis.

The radial nerve at the arcade of Frohse contains only motor fibers, except for those of the distal posterior interosseous nerve supplying propioceptive fibers to the dorsal wrist capsule; therefore, a sensory deficit should not be expected. Compression will only cause loss of active finger extension, as wrist extensors are innervated more proximally. Inability to actively extend the fingers can be confused with a tendon rupture or dislocation of the tendons to the ulnar side of the metacarpophalangeal joints. Under normal circumstances, passive flexion and extension of the wrist causes opposite mobility at the metacarpopha-langeal joints from what it is known as a tenodesis effect. In the presence of radial nerve palsy the tenodesis maneuver can be reproduced, as the muscle–tendon unit remains intact. Differential diagnosis of a tendon rupture or dislocation will be discussed in the following section.

1.3. Tendon–muscle examination

Examination of the tendon–muscle unit is essential in the rheumatoid hand as it is the most important cause of deformities. Joint synovitis will destroy the stabilizing structures and the pull of the muscles will be responsible for the deformities.

Joint assessment can be done radiographically, but muscle function can only be assessed by careful clinical examination. Muscle tissue alterations are mainly those of atrophy due to the lack of use, and shortening or retraction after prolonged periods of immobilization.

Tendon synovitis is quite frequent in rheumatoid disease, causing pain, loss of gliding, adhesions and even ruptures. In the following sections, we will describe the clinical manifestations of tendon synovitis, ruptures, dislocations, elongations and imbalance leading to boutonnière and swan neck deformities of the fingers.

Although the intrinsic muscles are not directly affected by joint or tendon synovitis, they are frequently involved in the form of retraction.

1.3.1. Tendon synovitis

Tendons are enveloped by tenosynovium only as they course inside osteo-fibrous compartments. Tenosynovitis of the flexor tendons can present at the carpal tunnel or the digital flexor tendon sheath, and tenosynovitis of the extensor tendons only at the extensor retinaculum. Contrary to the above, any alteration of the extensor tendons at the level of the MP, PIP or DIP joints will be secondary to underlying joint synovitis.

Tenosynovitis inside the extensor retinaculum may involve all tendons crossing the six extensor compartments, although the most frequently diagnosed are those involving the finger extensors and the extensor carpi ulnaris tendons. Synovitis of the *extensor digitorum communis* tendons (EDC) is easily diagnosed after observing swelling at the dorsum of the wrist, proximal and distal to the *extensor retinaculum*, resulting in an hourglass deformity. Swelling is more prominent distal to the *retinaculum* because the dorsal skin and fascia of the hand are thinner than those of the forearm. This should not be confused with a wrist joint synovitis, as it is located deeper and its capsule is more difficult to distend. When asking the patient to flex and extend the MP joints of the fingers, the mass can be seen and palpated moving distally and proximally, respectively.

Tenosynovitis of the *extensor carpi ulnaris* (ECU) tendon can be diagnosed by palpation at the level of the sixth extensor compartment. The styloid process of the ulna can be palpated following the posterior crest of the ulna, in line with the olecranon process. The ECU tendon runs trough an osteo-fibrous compartment just lateral to the ulnar styloid, and its relation to the hand will vary depending if its exploration is done with the forearm in pronation or supination. With the forearm in pronation it will be palpated at the ulnar side of the wrist. Elongation of the *extensor retinaculum* will cause anterior dislocation of the ECU tendon as most hand activities are done with the forearm in pronation. Volar translocation and supination of the carpus will increase the forces causing subluxation of the tendon.

Tenosynovitis of the finger flexor tendons inside the carpal tunnel is more difficult to diagnose as the overlying structures are more difficult to distend. However, looking at the distal forearm, we can observe a loss of concavity normally present just proximal to the wrist joint crease. The bulging tenosynovium can be palpated and felt to move proximally and distally when the patient actively flexes and extends the fingers.

Tenosynovitis inside the flexor tendon sheath can be diagnosed by palpation of the volar aspect of the finger, which will be enlarged. Flexor tendon synovitis may cause triggering and pain when flexing the finger, loss of active interphalangeal flexion and a swan neck deformity in long-standing cases [1]. Tenosynovitis of the flexor tendons is diagnosed by asking the patient to flex the IP joints while applying some pressure over the tendon just proximal to the A1 pulley of the flexor tendon sheath. The patient will experience discomfort, and the examining person will notice swelling, grinding and mild triggering from the hypertrophic synovium going in and out of the flexor tendon sheath. Definite diagnosis is made when the patient cannot fully flex the IP joints actively, while full passive flexion is possible (Fig. 1A and B).

1.3.2. Tendon ruptures

Examination is done by asking the patient to move the joint in the direction of pull of the muscle to be examined.

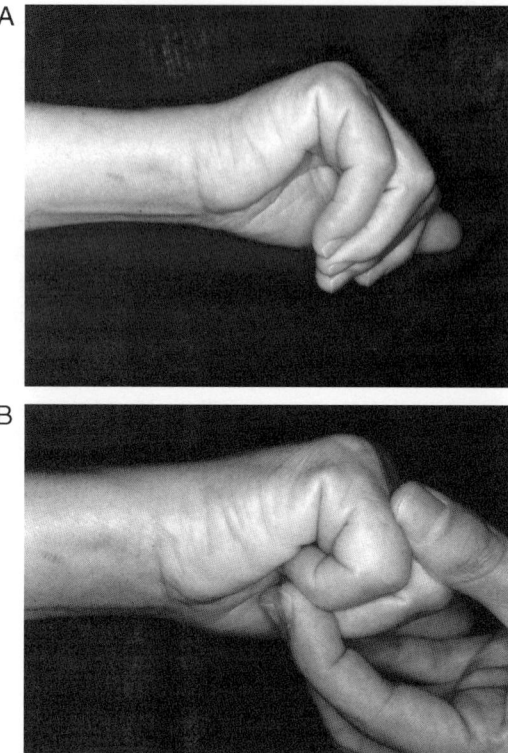

Fig. 1. (A) Patients with tenosynovitis of the flexor tendons inside the digital flexor tendon sheath will be unable to completely flex the interphalangeal joints. (B) Full passive interphalangeal joint flexion will rule out joint stiffness as a cause of loss of active finger flexion.

Integrity of wrist motors can be assessed by asking the patient to extend and flex the wrist. Radial and ulnar inclinations should be examined with the forearm in pronation and supination; as the extensor carpi ulnaris extends the wrist in supination and inclines it towards the ulnar side when the forearm is placed in pronation. Loss of wrist extension can be secondary to severe joint deformity or ankylosis. Wrist extensors may rupture as they cross the second extensor compartment of the wrist. Hypertrophic tendon synovitis at this level may cause rupture of tendon fibers from both ischemia and collagen fiber weakening from the surrounding inflamed synovium. However, the most important factor is tendon friction against the distal end of the radius, as most tendon ruptures are observed in cases of severe anterior translocation of the carpus. Contrary to finger extensor tendons, rupture of wrist extensors does not cause sudden loss of joint extension, as the wrist can still be extended from the pull of the intact finger extensors. Diagnosis of *extensor carpi radialis longus* (ECRL) and *brevis* (ECRB) tendon ruptures will be made in those cases in which passive wrist extension is greater than active extension. Many times, a definite diagnosis of wrist extensor rupture cannot be made until dorsal wrist surgery is performed, in which case one can observe the tendon gap bridged by scarred tissue which will provide some degree of active wrist extension.

Rupture of the *flexor carpi radialis* (FCR) tendon may occur inside the osteo-fibrous compartment at the distal scaphoid and trapezium, although its diagnosis may be overlooked as wrist flexion and can also be provided by the powerful finger flexors. A definite diagnosis can only be made by palpation of the tendon proximal to the wrist flexion crease during muscle contraction.

Integrity of the *flexor digitorum profundus* tendons (FDP) can be assessed by asking the patient to fully flex the fingers. If the fingers do not flex at the interphalangeal joints, it may be due to a flexor tendon rupture, interphalangeal joint stiffness or flexor tendon synovitis. Full passive interphalangeal joint flexion will rule out a joint problem, and either tendon synovitis or rupture will be the cause of loss of active finger flexion. In the presence of a flexor tendon rupture, the finger will be completely flail in extension, and in cases of flexor tendon synovitis or tendon adhesions, the finger will be moderately flexed and a certain degree of active finger flexion can be felt.

Integrity of the *flexor digitorum superficialis* tendons (FDS) is not routinely examined by many physicians, but it should be done in the manner which will be explained later. Although innervated by both the median and ulnar nerves, all fibers of the FDP muscle contract at the same time and actively flex the distal interphalangeal joints of all fingers. Only the fibers of the FDP to the index finger can contract somewhat independently from the rest. On the other hand, the FDS muscle, entirely innervated by the median nerve, has independent fibers for each finger, and flexes the finger at the proximal interphalangeal (PIP) joint. When the patient is asked to flex each individual finger, while the rest of the fingers are held in full extension by the examining physician, he will only be able to flex the finger at the PIP joint from contraction of the FDS muscle. The examination is done first with the ring finger, followed by the middle, small and index fingers (Fig. 2A). The FDS tendon will be ruptured if the patient cannot flex the finger being examined, while the rest of the fingers are kept in extension (Fig. 2B). Inability to flex the PIP joint of the small finger does not mean necessarily that the FDS has ruptured, as in many patients the FDS of the small finger is almost non existent or contracts together with that of the ring finger. In these cases, the PIP joint of the small finger will flex together with the one of the ring finger if the latter is allowed to be flexed. As mentioned previously, the FDP of the index finger can be somewhat independent from the rest and provide some finger flexion even if the rest of the fingers are kept in extension. Powerful contraction may cause some pain or discomfort in the forearm, and for this reason it should be examined last.

The exact location of a finger flexor tendon rupture may be hard to determine, as rupture may occur either at the carpal tunnel or inside the digital flexor tendon sheath [2]. The *flexor pollicis longus* (FPL) and the FDP tendon to the index finger are the tendons most commonly ruptured, usually from abrasion and wear against a prominent bony spicule of the flexed scaphoid which has eroded through the volar wrist capsule [3]. Flexor tendon ruptures inside the digital flexor tendon sheath almost always are secondary to infiltrative tenosynovitis [4]. FDS tendons rarely rupture at the carpal canal, as they are not located close to bony prominences of the carpal bones. FDS tendons rupture more frequently inside the flexor tendon sheath, probably because they split into two slips, diminishing their cross-sectional area by half, and also from increasing their surface of contact with the invading synovium, usually more prominent near the *vincula tendinum* at the distal third of the proximal phalanx.

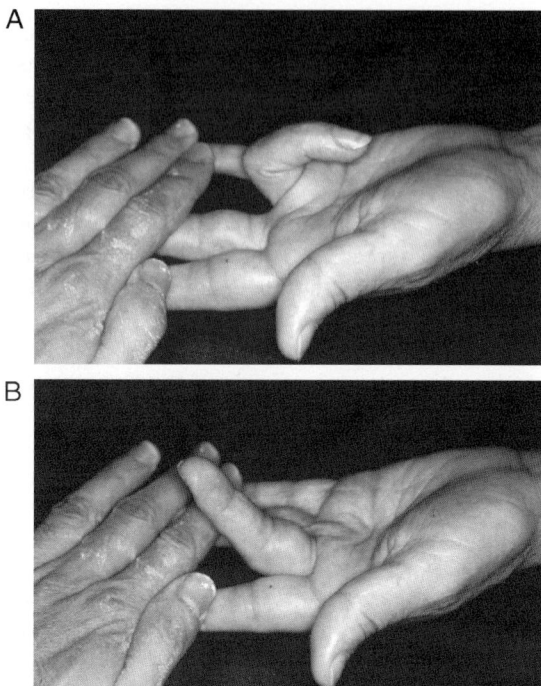

Fig. 2. (A) While keeping the fingers in extension, the patient is able to flex the PIP joint of the ring finger from contraction of the FDS muscle, demonstrating integrity of the FDS tendon. Some flexion at the DIP joint can be observed from adhesions between the FDS and the FDP tendons. (B) The patient is unable to flex the PIP joint of the middle finger, indicating rupture of the FDS tendon.

Rupture of FDS tendons are frequently overlooked, because the patient can still fully flex the finger, and exploration for individual FDS function is not done routinely. Palpating the volar aspect of the finger and finding an empty sheath, usually at the level of the proximal phalanx, will establish the level of rupture.

Integrity of the *flexor pollicis longus* (FPL) is tested by asking the patient to flex the interphalangeal (IP) joint of the thumb. Examination can be difficult in cases in which the IP joint is stiff in extension, usually associated to a severe flexion deformity of the metacarpophalangeal (MP) joint. FPL tendon rupture is usually secondary to friction against the distal end of a severely flexed scaphoid.

Integrity of the *extensor pollicis longus* (EPL) is assessed by asking the patient to extend the IP joint of the thumb. Since the IP joint can also be extended by contraction of the thenar muscles, the best way to determine the contractility of the EPL muscle is by asking the patient to place the thumb into retropulsion, and in particular in those cases in which the IP joint of the thumb is stiff in extension. EPL tendon rupture occurs at the third extensor compartment from friction against Lister's tubercle.

Contraction of the *extensor digitorum* muscle (EDC) extends the fingers at the MP joints. If the patient is unable to extend the MP joints, it may be secondary to any of the following causes: tendon rupture, tendon dislocation towards the ulnar side of the MP joint or posterior interosseous nerve (PIN) compression. In the presence of PIN compression, all the fingers will be affected at the same time, and some degree of MP joint extension can be obtained from a tenodesis effect by flexing the wrist, as the muscle–tendon unit remains intact. On the other hand, tendon rupture usually is sequential, starting first in the most ulnar fingers, as they rupture from friction against the head of the ulna, which is seen dorsally dislocated [5]. When the tendon ruptures, the patient experiences a sudden loss of finger extension and most times a "snap" and pain at the wrist level. In such cases, an ulnar translocation of the carpal bones can also be observed, as this causes displacement of the finger extensor tendons towards the head of the ulna [6].

1.3.3. Tendon dislocation, elongation and imbalance

Progressive ulnar drift of the fingers is one of the most characteristic deformities of the rheumatoid hand, which is generally secondary to ulnar dislocation of the extensor tendons towards the ulnar side of the MP joints.

The finger extensor tendons are stabilized at the dorsum of the metacarpal heads by two aponeurotic expansions, named sagittal bands, which insert at both sides of the volar plate of the MP joint. The sagittal bands are responsible for maintaining the extensor tendon at the dorsum of the joint while performing radial and ulnar inclination of the fingers, as well as allowing them to glide distally and proximally during joint flexion and extension. Synovitis of the MP joints will attenuate the sagittal bands, allowing the extensor tendons to dislocate towards the ulnar side. As long as the extensor tendon is maintained dorsal to the axis of rotation of the joint the patient will be able to actively extend the MP joint, but this will increase the forces causing further ulnar inclination of the fingers (Fig. 3).

If the dislocated extensor tendon falls below the axis of rotation of the joint, active extension will be impossible (Fig. 4). A differential diagnosis should be made between a tendon rupture and a posterior interosseous nerve compression. During the early stages, the ulnar sagittal band will not have had time to remodel in a shortened position and the

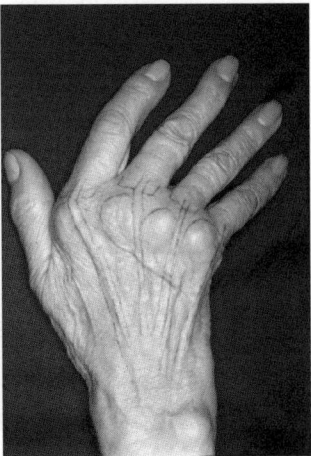

Fig. 3. Ulnar drift of the fingers caused by dislocation of the extensor tendons towards the ulnar side of the metacarpal heads.

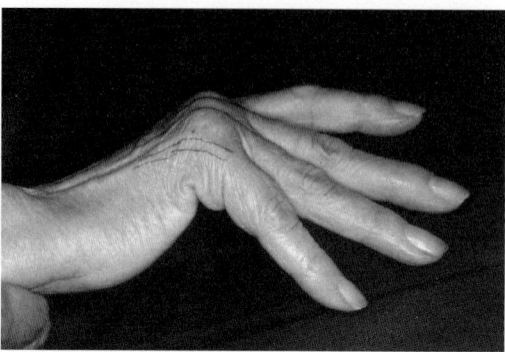

Fig. 4. The patient is unable to extend the MP joints because the extensor tendon has dislocated and displaced anterior to the axis of joint rotation.

extensor tendon will be maintained at the dorsum of the joint by contraction of the finger extensor muscle after the finger is passively placed in extension (Fig. 5). When the patient stops extensor muscle contraction the finger will drop again into flexion because the radial sagittal band has been elongated and therefore unable to maintain the tendon at the dorsum of the joint.

As time passes, the ulnar sagittal band will remodel in a shortened position and the previous manoeuvre cannot be reproduced. Contraction of the extensor tendon muscle will then cause MP joint flexion, as well as ulnar inclination and some degree of finger rotation into supination. If we passively correct the finger deformity and maintain it in this position, we will find that the finger flexes, supinates and goes into ulnar inclination when the patient is asked to contract the finger extensor muscle. The extensor tendons can also be seen and palpated at the dorsum of the wrist, ruling out an extensor tendon rupture.

Synovitis of the PIP joints will cause attenuation of the extensor apparatus and progressive loss of active joint extension. In normal circumstances, when the PIP joint is in full extension, both the central slip and the lateral bands are located dorsal to the axis of rotation of the joint, assisting together to extend the joint. As the PIP joint flexes, the

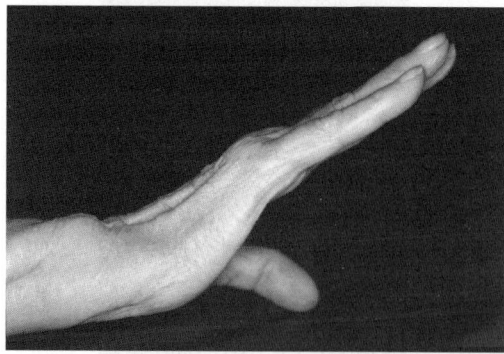

Fig. 5. If the MP joints are passively extended, the patient can maintain the fingers in this position by contraction of the extensor tendon muscle. This can only be observed in the early stages of the deformity, before the ulnar sagittal band remodels in a shortened position preventing dorsal relocation of the extensor tendons.

lateral bands displace to the sides of the joint to allow DIP joint flexion. The central slip and the lateral bands are held together by a thin layer of connective tissue which allows some lateral and longitudinal displacement of the latter during joint flexion. The loss of active PIP joint extension is not only from attenuation of the central slip but also from progressive volar displacement of the lateral bands, as the hypertrophic joint synovitis will attenuate the connective tissue holding the lateral bands and the central slip together. Under these circumstances, the extensor apparatus will displace proximally causing extension of the DIP joint. Flexion of the PIP joint together with extension of the DIP joint is known as *boutonnière* or *button-hole deformity*, as the condyles of the proximal phalanx are seen protruding dorsally in between the lateral bands just as a button through a buttonhole. Extension of the MP joint has also been described as part of a boutonnière deformity, but this will only be seen when the patient can extend the MP joint in order to place the tip of the finger aligned with the palm of the hand. We can observe many boutonnière deformities with a flexion deformity of the MP joint.

Nalebuff and Millender [7] have presented a useful classification for the surgical treatment of boutonnière deformities. In stage I, the patient has only a slight loss of active PIP joint extension. The joint can be passively extended and there is minimal hyperextension deformity of the DIP joint. In stage II, the PIP joint is moderately flexed, from 30° to 40°, and the DIP joint is extended, although some passive correction can be obtained. In stage III, the deformity in both interphalangeal joints cannot be passively corrected (Fig. 6).

When examining the PIP joint we should determine the presence of joint synovitis, which is easily seen and palpated bulging dorsally and proximally underneath the extensor apparatus. In many cases, after careful clinical examination, and specially during surgical exploration, we can see a herniation of the hypertrophic synovium in between the central slip and lateral bands.

Next, we should asses if the PIP joint flexion contracture can be corrected. This should be done by applying pressure to the middle phalanx, leaving the DIP joint free. If the DIP

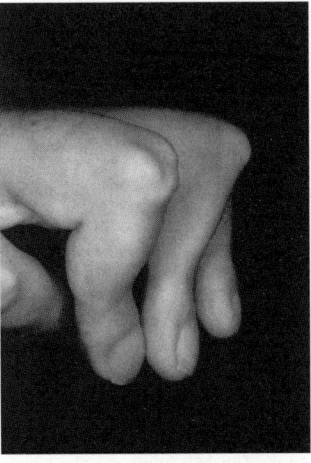

Fig. 6. Boutonnière deformity of the fingers. The PIP joints are flexed and the DIP joint are extended.

joint hyperextension corrects by itself after passively extending the PIP joint, it is because the lateral bands move back again to the dorsum of the PIP joint. If the lateral bands do not displace dorsally, from retraction of the transverse retinaculars ligament, passive PIP joint extension will not correct and may even worsen the hyperextension deformity of the DIP joint.

If the PIP joint cannot be passively extended at all, a radiographic examination should be done to rule out joint destruction.

Swan-neck deformities have also been classified in four stages by Nalebuff [8]. In stage I, the PIP joint is flexible in all positions, including MP joint extension. In stage II, the PIP joint cannot be fully flexed if the MP joint is placed in extension, demonstrating intrinsic muscle tightness. In stage III, the PIP joint cannot be flexed even with MP joint flexion, demonstrating that loss of joint flexion is due to shortening of the extensor apparatus and the dorsal capsule. In stage IV, the PIP joint is also stiff in extension but radiographic examination shows signs of joint destruction or an ankylosis.

Contrary to boutonnière deformities, swan-neck deformities may cause a fixed deformity of the MP joint. The MP joint will present with a flexion contracture from shortening of the intrinsic muscles (Fig. 7).

1.3.4. Intrinsic muscle examination

Intrinsic muscle tightness is frequently seen in the rheumatoid hand. It has been postulated that this could be secondary to "spasticity" or "irritation" from synovitis at the MP joints, but the fact is that intrinsic muscle tightness can be seen even in hands without MP joint synovitis. Intrinsic muscle retraction is a physiological shortening of the muscle sarcomere, occurring in any muscle, after its origin and insertion have been approximated for prolonged periods of time. This will occur after prolonged MP joint flexion, quite frequent in the rheumatoid hand from loss of active joint extension. The ulnar intrinsic muscles can be seen more retracted in cases of ulnar drift of the fingers.

The intrinsic muscles originate at the metacarpal bones and insert into the proximal phalanx and the extensor apparatus. Their main function is flexing the MP joints, although their insertion into the extensor apparatus provides extension of the PIP

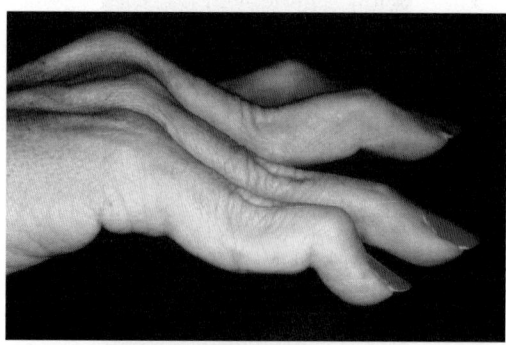

Fig. 7. Swan neck deformity of the fingers. The MP joints are flexed, the PIP joints are extended and the DIP joints are flexed.

joints. From a mechanical point of view, their line of pull is volarly located in relation to the axis of rotation of the MP joint and dorsally located to the axis of rotation of the PIP joint.

Under normal circumstances, PIP joint flexion can be accomplished with the MP joint fully extended due to the elasticity of the muscle fibres. If the intrinsic muscles are remodelled in a shorter position, PIP joint flexion will be limited as MP joint extension increases. Ulnar and radial intrinsics should be explored for shortening by placing the MP joint in extension and in radial and ulnar inclinations respectively. The ulnar intrinsics are usually shorter than the radial intrinsics secondary to a long standing ulnar drift of the fingers (Fig. 8).

In cases of severe intrinsic muscle retraction, extension of the MP joints will not be possible. This will be due to intrinsic muscle tightness, as well as secondary shortening of capsular structures of the MP joint and even skin shortening. All above alterations should be assessed, as a successful correction of a swan-neck deformity depends on the correction of all abnormalities, including release of flexor tendon adhesions, which are always present in longstanding deformities [1].

In cases of ulnar drift of the fingers, the radial intrinsics will become weak and atrophy from lack of use. This becomes more evident when exploring the first dorsal interosseous muscle. Radial intrinsic muscle weakness is an added factor to explain a recurrence of ulnar drift of the fingers after surgical correction (Fig. 9).

1.4. Joint examination

When examining a joint, the following should be observed:

1. Presence and intensity of joint swelling, from joint fluid and hypertrophic synovitis.
2. Attenuation or complete rupture of ligaments, assessed by passive testing of joint stability.

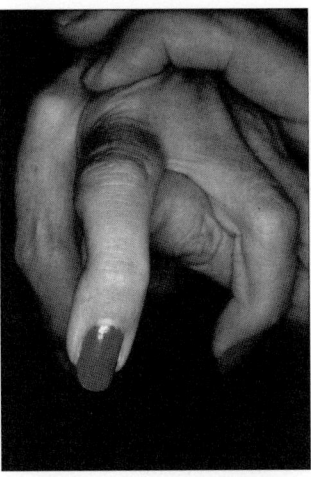

Fig. 8. When the MP joint is placed in extension and the ulnar inclination is corrected, the PIP joint cannot be flexed, neither actively or passively, indicating retraction of the ulnar intrinsic muscle.

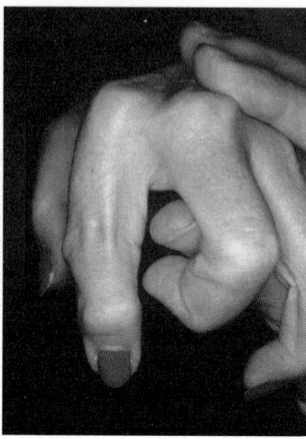

Fig. 9. If the same finger is examined with ulnar inclination of the MP joint, PIP joint flexion will be possible, demonstrating ulnar intrinsic tightness and absence of radial intrinsic shortening.

3. Posture at rest, secondary to tendon imbalance. Tendon imbalance can be secondary to tendon elongation, tendon rupture or tendon dislocation. Tendons undergoing subluxation will cross the axis of joint rotation at an abnormal angle, causing a joint deformity in the direction of the muscle pull. With time, muscle fiber retraction will prevent the joint from being passively corrected in the opposite direction. Later on, capsular structures will be remodeled in a shortened position, further preventing passive joint correction.
4. Grinding test to determine degree of joint cartilage destruction.

The intensity of joint synovitis and that of joint deformity, destruction or stiffness are not always parallel, and my not coincide simultaneously. In the early stages of the disease, we can observe important joint synovitis without joint deformity. On the contrary, during the later stages of the disease, joint deformity and destruction may be more pronounced, while joint synovitis will tend to resolve from decreased joint mobility or ankylosis.

Apart from recording the existence and degree of joint deformities observed at rest, we should also explore the active range of joint mobility. Finally, we should determine if the deformities are passively corrected, being careful not to cause unnecessary discomfort to the patient [9]. Using a goniometer, the range of motion should be recorded according to the neutral-zero position, following the guidelines recommended by the International Federation of Societies for Surgery of the Hand [10].

The last thing that we would like to find out about the wrist joint is its degree of stiffness, first described by Clayton [11] and later by Simmen and Huber [12], as this implies important therapeutic considerations. This can be assessed by passively displacing the wrist in the antero-posterior plane and observing the amount of instability secondary to the degree of ligament and bone destruction.

In the following sections we will describe the most common deformities in the different joints of the hand.

1.4.1. The wrist joint

The wrist consists of 14 individual joints which, from the functional point of view, can be grouped into three main joints: radiocarpal, midcarpal and distal radioulnar. The distal radioulnar joint is designed to provide rotation of the distal radius around the ulnar head, allowing for pronation and supination of the forearm and hand. While extension, flexion, radial and ulnar inclinations of the wrist take place at the radiocarpal and midcarpal joints.

Because the joint surface of the distal radius presents an anterior inclination of approximately 10° and an ulnar inclination of approximately 23°, the forces transmitted by the wrist and finger flexor muscles will tend to displace the carpal bones into an anterior and ulnar direction. To prevent this, the radiocarpal ligaments are obliquely oriented, running from radial-proximal to distal-ulnar.

Joint synovitis will cause capsular and ligament attenuation, and the forces acting through the joint will be responsible for the deformities. We will describe the deformities in the 3 main functional joints of the wrist.

1.4.1.1. The radiocarpal and midcarpal joints.

Radiocarpal joint synovitis will cause ligament destruction, which will be responsible for a progressive displacement of the carpal bones towards the ulnar side. Although the deforming forces are mainly in an anterior direction, anterior translation of the carpus is less commonly observed because the radio–lunate joint is more constrained in this plane due to the concavity of the distal radius, and similar radius of curvature of the radius and the lunate bone. Only in cases with acute and intense joint synovitis, causing severe ligament destruction, will the carpus be completely dislocated anteriorly, with the possibility of displacing the lunate bone a few centimetres proximal to the anterior edge of the distal radius.

The midcarpal joint is more constrained, and therefore deformities at this level are less important than at the radiocarpal joint.

1.4.1.2. The distal radioulnar joint (DRUJ).

DRUJ synovitis is very common in rheumatoid disease, causing attenuation of the radioulnar and ulnocarpal ligaments. Synovitis is easily palpable on the dorsal and ulnar sides of the joint. Attenuation of the radioulnar ligaments will cause instability of the DRUJ. We can asses the degree of instability by passive displacement of the ulnar head in relation to the radius. This exploration should be done with the forearm in neutral position, as the DRUJ becomes more stable in the extremes of pronation and supination. With further destruction of the distal radioulnar ligaments, dorsal dislocation of the distal ulna can be observed, mainly when placing the forearm in pronation [13]. In the majority of cases, forearm supination may be limited.

Destruction of the ulnocarpal ligaments, ulno-lunate, ulno-triquetral and ulno-capitate, will cause the ulnar side of the carpus to displace anteriorly due to the forces transmitted by the finger flexors and the flexor carpi ulnaris tendons. The ECU tendon may also contribute to the deformity in those cases where it is dislocated anteriorly from its compartment on the ulnar head. This will cause a supination deformity of the carpus, which clinically will appear more severe due to the concomitant dorsal displacement of the distal ulna [14]. Frequent involvement of the distal radioulnar joint will be responsible for the loss of ulnar buttress to the carpus provided by the triangular fibrocartilaginous complex (TFCC), and therefore is another reason why we see a greater ulnar rather than anterior displacement of the carpus in many rheumatoid wrists.

In summarizing, rheumatoid arthritis can cause the following deformities at the wrist: ulnar translocation, anterior displacement, supination deformity and ulnar inclination. A comment should be made about the radial and ulnar inclination of the wrist. Following an observation made by Jules Shapiro in 1970 [15], it is commonly stated that wrist joint synovitis causes a radial inclination of the metacarpals. However, the truth is that wrist joint synovitis, regardless of its aetiology, will always deviate the wrist towards the ulnar side. The radial inclination commonly observed in the rheumatoid hand is secondary to the ulnar inclination of the fingers at the metacarpophalangeal joint level. This is a volitional deformity, produced by the patient, in an attempt to align the fingers with the longitudinal axis of the forearm, to obtain a better digital function as well as appearance [6,14,16,17]. The same can be observed after fractures of the distal end of the radius which have healed with a loss of the normal volar or ulnar inclination of the distal joint surface. Under these circumstances, the patient will always place his wrist in a direction opposite to the bone deformity, with the purpose of aligning the fingers with the longitudinal axis of the forearm. In conclusion, when only the wrist is involved by the disease it will always deviate towards the ulnar side.

1.4.2. The MP joints

Persistent synovitis of the metacarpophalangeal (MP) joints destroys the collateral ligaments, and the proximal phalanx progressively displaces anteriorly from the pull of the intrinsic and extrinsic flexor muscles. Integrity of the collateral ligaments is explored with full MP joint flexion. In this position and under normal circumstances, ulnar and radial inclination of the proximal phalanx will not be possible as the ligaments are placed under tension. In the rheumatoid patient, we can observe a radioulnar instability of the joint even in early stages, before volar subluxation occurs. Later on we can see an increased passive displacement of the proximal phalanx in the anteroposterior plane, similar to the "drawer" sign used for exploring an anterior cruciate ligament rupture in the knee. In more advanced cases, if we look at the fingers from the side we can find an anterior subluxation of the proximal phalanx, some times masked by the dorsal hypertrophic synovitis. If the collateral ligaments and the sagittal bands are completely elongated, we can observe the heads of the metacarpals protruding under the skin, dorsal to the proximal phalanx. This deformity can be passively made more evident by pushing the proximal phalanx anteriorly.

The sagittal bands, which maintain the extensor tendon at the dorsum of the metacarpal head during flexion and extension of the joint, will also become attenuated. Due to an imbalance of forces towards the ulnar side, the radial sagittal band will progressively elongate, allowing for the extensor tendon to displace towards the ulnar side of the metacarpal head [18]. Ulnar deviation of the proximal phalanx is more frequently observed and more pronounced in the small finger, with decreasing incidence and deformity towards the more radial fingers. When the extensor tendon is markedly dislocated, the patient will not be able to actively extend the finger. If the tendon falls below the axis of rotation of the joint, its contraction will further flex the finger rather than extend it. When the patient is unable to actively extend the MP joints, the clinician should determine if it is due to a tendon rupture, a tendon dislocation or a muscle palsy secondary to a compression of the posterior interosseous nerve.

1.4.3. The PIP joints

Synovitis of the PIP joint will attenuate the central slip of the extensor apparatus, resulting in a loss of active extension of the joint. The lateral bands normally displace to the sides of the condyles of the proximal phalanx during joint flexion. As the joint progressively flexes, the loose connective tissue holding the lateral bands to the central slip will also elongate, increasing the anterior displacement of the lateral bands. With time, all extension forces on the PIP joint will be lost, progressively increasing the flexion deformity of the joint. The proximal displacement of the extensor apparatus will cause a hyperextension deformity of the DIP joint, creating a deformity known as boutonnière.

If the collateral ligaments become attenuated, a lateral instability of the joint, as well as a volar displacement of the middle phalanx, will occur.

1.4.4. The DIP joints

Synovitis of the DIP joints will attenuate the distal extensor tendon, resulting in a loss of the extension forces upon the joint. The contraction of the flexor digitorum profundus tendon will be responsible for a flexion deformity of the joint, known as *mallet finger deformity*.

We should measure the degree of the deformity, as well as recording its passive correction if possible.

2. Plain radiographic examination

Radiographic examination should always be done to determine the degree of joint cartilage damage, as deformities with joint damage should not be treated by soft tissue rebalancing but rather by artrodesis or arthroplasty.

The most frequently used method for grading joint destruction is the one described by Larsen et al. [19].

Apart from the progressive degrees of joint destruction described by Larsen et al., different patrons of cartilage and bone destruction can be observed. Some type of synovitis, usually low grade, will destroy the joint cartilage with little joint deformity, and present with radiographic signs similar to those of a degenerative arthritis. Other types of synovitis, usually very acute and intense, may cause a rapid rupture of the stabilizing ligaments resulting in a complete dislocation of the joint with minimal or no cartilage destruction. Less frequently, we can observe joints with severe bone resorption causing an arthritis mutilans type of deformity, known as "opera-glass hand" [20] when it involves the fingers. This type of destruction is mainly observed at the MP joints, causing what has been named as a "pencil and cup deformity" [21], characterised by resorption and thinning the metacarpal head articulating against a moderately resorbed and widened proximal phalangeal end.

In the presence of a fixed joint, radiographic examination should be done to rule out the existence of joint ankylosis.

We should measure the degree of ulnar translocation of the carpus on an anterior posteroanterior radiograph of the wrist, using one of the different methods proposed [22–24]. On the lateral view, we can measure the anterior translocation of the carpus [25].

3. Computed axial tomography (CAT scan)

CAT scan examination can be most useful to asses the deformities at the wrist, as simple radiographic examination, due to the osteoporotic characteristics of the bone as well as the severe deformities in some cases, will make its interpretation very difficult. The scaphoid can be flexed 90°, while the lunate seems to have disappeared. The lunate either can be found at the volar and ulnar side of the distal radius or even be impacted inside the distal radius through a very thin subchondral bone.

Volar subluxation of the proximal phalanx is often accompanied with a "scalloping" deformity of its dorsal aspect from impaction against the head of the metacarpal. Important loss of the proximal and dorsal phalangeal cortex has therapeutic implications when planning the type of joint arthroplasty to be used. This can be assessed by careful radiographic examination in both anteroposterior and true lateral views (Fig. 10). CAT scan examination will better demonstrate the deformity.

4. Magnetic resonance imaging (MRI)

The presence of wrist joint synovitis is difficult to determine on clinical examination, as it is located deep under the extensor and flexor muscles and its capsule is not easily distended. MRI examination will demonstrate synovitis at the radiocarpal, midcarpal and distal radioulnar joints in its early stages (Fig. 11).

MRI examination will also clearly demonstrate the presence, extend and amount of tendon synovitis either at the wrist or at the fingers.

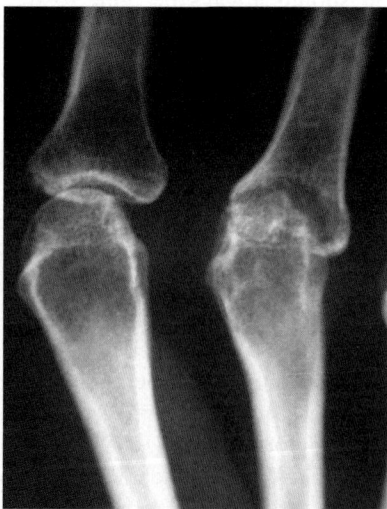

Fig. 10. Posteroanterior radiograph shows subluxation of the MP joint of the index finger and dorsal cortical erosion, "scalloping", of the proximal phalanx of the middle finger.

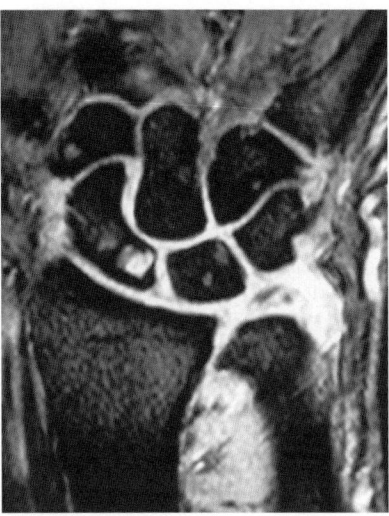

Fig. 11. MRI examination of the wrist demonstrating hypertrophic synovitis of DRUJ and radiocarpal joints.

MRI examination may also help in determining the location of a tendon rupture.

5. Bone scan examination

Bone scan examination is seldom used in the rheumatoid patient, except in those cases in which early joint synovitis is suspected, mainly at the wrist joint. It can also be used to determine the number of possible multiple joint involvement in patients seen at first with symptoms in a single joint.

References

[1] A. Lluch, The treatment of finger joint deformities in rheumatoid arthritis, in: Y. Allieu (Ed.), The Rheumatoid Hand and Wrist, Expansion Scientifique Publications, Paris, 1998, pp. 85–104.
[2] D.C. Ferlic, Rheumatoid flexor tenosynovitis and rupture, Hand Clin. 12 (1996) 561–572.
[3] N. Mannerfelt, O. Norman, Attrition ruptures of flexor tendons in rheumatoid arthritis caused by bony spurs in the carpal tunnel, J. Bone Jt. Surg. 51B (1969) 270–277.
[4] A.N. Ertel, et al., Flexor tendon ruptures in patients with rheumatoid arthritis, J. Hand Surg. 13A (1988) 860–866.
[5] O.J. Vaughan-Jackson, Rupture of extensor tendons by attrition at the inferior radio-ulnar joint. Report of two cases, J. Bone Jt. Surg. 30B (1948) 528–530.
[6] A. Lluch, Aspects actuels du poignet rhumatoïde, in: J. Duparc (Ed.), Cahiers d'Enseignement de la SOFCOT, Elsevier, Amsterdam, 2000, pp. 203–221.
[7] E.A. Nalebuff, C.H. Millender, Surgical treatment of the boutonniere deformity in rheumatoid arthritis, Orthop. Clin. North Am. 6 (1975) 753–763.
[8] E.A. Nalebuff, The rheumatoid swan-neck deformity, Hand Clin. 5 (1989) 203–214.
[9] D. Herren, B.R. Simmen, Rheumatoid arthritis of the wrist, in: R.A. Berger, A.-P.C. Weiss (Eds.), Hand Surg., Lippincott Williams & Wilkins, Philadelphia, 2004, pp. 1213–1240.
[10] I. Leslie, A. Lluch (Eds.), Terminology for Hand Surgery. IFSSH, Harcourt Health Sciences, London, 2001.
[11] M.L. Clayton, Surgical treatment at the wrist in rheumatoid arthritis. A review of thirty-seven patients, J. Hand Surg. 47-A (1965) 741–750.

[12] B.R. Simmen, H. Huber, The rheumatoid wrist: a new classification related to the type of the natural course and its consequences for surgical therapy, in: B. Simmen, F.-W. Hagena (Eds.), The Wrist in Rheumatoid Arthritis, Karger, Basel, 1992, pp. 13–25.

[13] M. Backdahl, The caput ulnae syndrome in rheumatoid arthritis: a study of the morphology, abnormal anatomy and clinical picture, Acta Rheumatol. Scand. 5 (1963) 1–75.

[14] E. Zancolli, The wrist and the metacarpal arch in rheumatoid arthritis – the supination collapse of the hand, Hand Surg. 1 (1996) 219–237.

[15] J.S. Shapiro, A new factor in the aetiology of ulnar drift, Clin. Orthop. 68 (1970) 32–43.

[16] A. Lluch, Surgery for the rheumatoid wrist, in: A. Renner (Ed.), 9th Congress of the IFSSH. International Proceedings, Bologna, Medimond, 2004, pp. 39–46.

[17] A.E. Flatt, Ulnar drift, in: A.E. Flatt (Ed.), The Care of the Rheumatoid Hand, Fifth edition, Quality Medical Publishing Inc., St. Louis, 1995, p. 346.

[18] A. Lluch, Metacarpophalangeal arthroplasties, in: J. Duparc (Ed.), Surgical Techniques in Orthopaedics and Traumatology, Elsevier, Paris, 2000, pp. 1–5, 55-320-C-10.

[19] A. Larsen, K. Dale, M. Eek, Radiographic evaluation of rheumatoid arthritis and related condition by standard reference films, Acta Radiol., Diagn. 18 (1976) 481–491.

[20] E.A. Nalebuff, J. Garret, Opera-glass hand in rheumatoid arthritis, J. Hand Surg. 1 (1976) 210–220.

[21] O.J. Vaughan-Jackson, Egg-cup erosion, Hand 1 (1969) 9–13.

[22] H.-W. Bouman, E. Messer, G. Sennwald, Measurement of ulnar translation and carpal height, J. Hand Surg. 19-B&E (1994) 325–329.

[23] M.R. DiBenedetto, L.M. Lubbers, C.R. Coleman, A standardized measurement of ulnar carpal translocation, J. Hand Surg. 15-A: 1009–1010.

[24] M.A. Pirela-Cruz, K. Firoozbakshsh, M.S. Moneim, Ulnar translation of the carpus in rheumatoid arthritis: an analysis of five determination methods, J. Hand Surg. 18-A (1993) 299–306.

[25] A. Pagliei, et al., Palmar subluxation of the carpus in rheumatoid disease: a radiological evaluation, Ann. Hand Surg. 10 (1991) 541–555.

International Congress Series 1295 (2006) 27–33

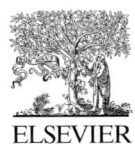

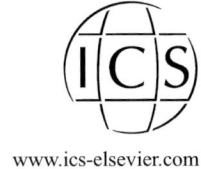

www.ics-elsevier.com

The timing of surgery in rheumatoid arthritis

John Stanley

Wrightington, Wigan and Leigh NHS Trust, United Kingdom

Abstract. A very accurate preoperative assessment of both the functional and social implications of the patient's problems should be performed. This forms the basis upon which an opinion as to which surgical procedures would be of benefit in any given patient situation can be made. At the same time we have to take cognisance of the importance of various structures in the surgical hierarchy. These have been outlined: nerves, flexor tendons, wrists, thumbs, metacarpophalangeal joints, extensor tendons, proximal interphalangeal joints, and distal interphalangeal joints. It is important to bear in mind that each surgical procedure takes a finite recovery time and takes a little more out of the patients, particularly if they have had rheumatoid arthritis for many years and are perhaps less able to withstand repeated major surgical procedures. These patients have often had hip surgery, knee surgery, shoulder surgery, elbow surgery before they come to their hand and foot surgery. I think it is very important to ensure that patients are not overwhelmed by this mammoth list of surgical procedures that have been identified as being helpful. Composite surgery is beneficial to the patient who is developing "surgical fatigue" where thumb fusion, wrist fusion or replacement and metacarpophalangeal joint surgery may be combined if appropriate. © 2006 Published by Elsevier B.V.

Keywords: Functional assessment; Surgical hierarchy; Composite surgery

1. Introduction

The aphorism that rheumatoid arthritis is a whole-body lifetime incurable disease for which the treatment is medical and not surgical is well known to everybody. It is also recognised that it is a multi-system disease affecting heart, lungs, blood vessels, nerves, as well as the problems with joints, tendons and ligaments. Because of the widespread nature of rheumatoid disease and its affect upon individuals, there is almost always a requirement

E-mail address: jacqueline.hughes@wwl.nhs.uk.

0531-5131/ © 2006 Published by Elsevier B.V.
doi:10.1016/j.ics.2006.03.069

to assess each and every patient as an individual with unique problems. If one starts from that premise, then one can more accurately decide upon the problems that need to be resolved in that individual against the background of their disease and identify the surgical procedures that might achieve a functional improvement. It is also well recognised that the mere presence of deformity, although giving rise to some loss of faculty does not necessarily give rise to a significant disability. It is important to understand the difference of the following three terms: loss of faculty or impairment, disability and handicap. Whilst the World Health Organisation in 1982 defined those terms, there is a more recent definition that is a little less clear. Having said that there is no doubt that, the definition of loss of faculty or impairment is derived from those things that one can measure, such as range of motion, sensibility, power, stamina, etc.

Whereas disability is the effect of that particular loss of faculty upon the individual, for example, the loss of the dominant little finger in the majority of people would be seen as being a significant loss of faculty (15% of hand function) and a significant disability because it would narrow the hand, prevent power grasp of a normal degree and in general become a nuisance to people, but can be coped with. So the disability might just equate to the loss of faculty, whereas if one is a violinist for example then the loss of the non-dominant little finger does give rise to increased disability. The loss of the non-dominant little finger prevents playing of the violin completely and gives rise to a 100% occupational disability.

Therefore, the disability would be significantly greater for a non-dominant little finger loss than a dominant little finger loss in such people as professional musicians. This example is really to highlight that loss of faculty does not equate necessarily to disability. Handicap is the effect of the disability on the person within the community, for example the wheelchair user will have difficulty climbing stairs and will use ramps instead; this identifies the individual's handicap.

When using these definitions it is important to appreciate that rheumatoid patients will always have a loss of faculty, they always have a disability, which has crept up on them over quite a long period of time, but which has usually allowed them to make necessary small incremental adaptations to their life style with activity modification to a degree which allows them to achieve their goals. However, there may come a point in time when that degree of compromise and adaptation is no longer possible and the addition of gadgets and little modifications to the items around the home are finally insufficient to mask the disability that exists. Nevertheless, each patient has his/her own lifestyle and some patients are very active and like to continue handicrafts, such as knitting, sewing, and gardening, and do-it-yourself activities. Others have no desire to practice these and are comfortable living a simple life and doing simple jobs around the home. Therefore, a fairly detailed knowledge of the patient's capacity, wishes and demands are an essential part of the pre-operative assessment of the patient.

2. Pre-operative assessment

As we have tried to outline in the Introduction, patients seek advice about functional problems that affect them in their particular lives. Therefore, one must consider that each patient is a unique problem to be solved and requires a unique solution. A best practice is being aware of this before considering operating on rheumatoid patients in order to avoid a "cook book" approach to this problem. A full functional upper limb assessment should be part of the pre-operative work up of the patient and certainly be performed prior to any surgical planning.

The preference in our Unit is:

a. to have a one-on-one interview,
b. to perform a SODA, i.e. sequential occupational dexterity assessment, and
c. to perform other appropriate assessments before committing to a surgical treatment programme.

The problem of any protocol-driven assessment tool is of course very often the difficulty of validation; assessments, such as DASH (i.e. disabilities of the arm shoulder and hand), are not really sensitive enough to pick-up subtle changes in these patients. Nonetheless, it provides a good baseline against which to measure their disability in the medium to long term. Any assessment should include a detailed review of the patient's practical problems in order to maintain their independence of existence. This is the prime objective of the management of patients with rheumatoid disease. The activities of daily living form the bedrock upon which any assessment is performed and that is the ability to feed, dress, toilet and attend to personal hygiene. One might add the capacity to shop, cook, drive, and so on, but these are issues that need to be assessed prior to definitive surgery. Having completed the pre-operative assessment and identified the nature, degree and the priority of the functional problems, each individual surgical team will have its own repertoire of surgery and the experienced therapist will be able to identify what he or she thinks is an appropriate treatment for the problems for the individual.

3. Functional assessment

There is no doubt that having done the functional assessment this should be followed by a functional anatomical assessment, which is defined as:

a. What is the problem?
b. What is the cause of the problem?
c. What needs to be done to improve the function?
d. What priority do I give to these problems?
e. What are the post-operative limitations to the patients' capacity to remain independent?
f. What are the potential negative effects of my actions?

4. Anatomical assessment

There is a requirement to be aware of functional anatomy as opposed to simple topographical anatomy. Functional anatomy is the basis of the understanding of rheumatoid surgery; that is to say, it is crucial to maintain and improve function and recognise that function is a product of multiple anatomical structures acting in unison. Therefore, if one tries to turn a key in a lock it is not sufficient to be able to improve the appositional key-type pinch by surgery to the thumb and or index finger because although key-pinch maybe restored, the requirement to turn a key in the lock requires the capacity to undertake pronation and supination of the forearm. Therefore, it may be necessary for a patient who has that specific difficulty to undergo stabilization of the thumb, stabilization of the metacarpophalangeal joint of the index finger *and* surgery for distal radial ulnar joint problems. In light of this one has to look at the interaction of various joint and tendon problems within the hand and upper limb in order to identify these functional anatomical patterns. Having completed a pre-operative assessment, having looked at the functional anatomy and decided on the various surgical procedures that might be of benefit for a patient, it is now necessary to do other assessments.

5. Medical assessment

The importance of appreciating the medical status of the patient and their current medical treatment cannot be over emphasised and close liaison and cooperation between Rheumatologist and Surgeon is essential if treatment is to be best timed and effective. If the patient has an active on-going rheumatoid process, then surgery is highly inadvisable. If the patient has splinter haemorrhages, acute nodules, then there is the possibility that they have significant Vasculitis and any wound will not heal well in these circumstances. It may be that they have pericarditis or pneumonitis, which both can give rise to significant risks during anaesthesia and decisions have to be made as to whether the surgery, as proposed, can be performed with a local anaesthetic, a regional anaesthetic or does it have to be a general anaesthetic. After completing all of those assessments, the final assessment is the surgical one.

6. Psychological assessment

There is the psychological assessment, deciding whether a patient is capable of understand or tolerating often long and complex rehabilitation programmes.

7. Financial assessment

There is the financial aspect of it, i.e., is the patient still working and will taking them away from work for any period of time jeopardise their current employment? Is surgery essential at this time for this patient? Can it be delayed until a point in time where the disease process itself prevents them from continuing to work?

8. Surgical assessment

8.1. Surgical hierarchy

The decision to operate on the patient must be made within the context of the hierarchy of surgical procedures; the following list is advisory only.

1. Nerves: There is clear evidence that prolonged compression of nerves gives rise to intra-neural fibrosis and in turn a poor recovery from simple decompression. In the light of the fact that both median and ulnar nerves, and to a lesser extent the radial nerve are vulnerable to compression in rheumatoid arthritis, there is a clear requirement to

consider nerve compression syndromes as being perhaps the first priority within a surgical cascade. Clearly any surgical cascade has to take account of what is required, what is practical, what is desirable and so on, but in terms of having a problem with nerves that should take precedence over all other aspects of hand surgery, other than thrombosis of vessels, and ischemia, which is very rare.

2. Flexor tendons: The second step would be to consider the flexor tendons. Flexor tendons are at risk from chronic compression, and are vulnerable to prolonged compression and to attrition rupture over sharp bony spurs, Mannerfelt described this phenomenon at the scaphoid trapezoidal joint where the flexor pollicis longus, the flexor digitorum profundus and later the flexor digitorum superficialis to the index finger can be completely ruptured by this attrition affect. Equally, the flexor to the little finger as it rubs over irregular surfaces on the piso triquetrial joint can be subject to a similar effect. Therefore, given that prolonged flexor tenosynovitis causes stiffness in the finger joints, there is a requirement to consider flexor tendons at an early stage in any surgical cascade. Ruptures are very difficult to deal with and multiple ruptures almost impossible to deal with. Therefore, there is a strong argument for prophylactic surgery, that is to say having a fairly low trigger to considering flexor tenosynovectomy.

3. The wrist: Because the flexor tendons cross the wrist and the muscles exist in the forearm attached to the radius and ulna and, to some extent, the humerus, there is a clear issue when thinking about the wrist joint itself. A painful unstable wrist joint will diminish the effectiveness of any power that is generated in the forearm wishing to be transferred to the hand, through the tendons. Therefore one should consider the wrist joint as being the third priority within the hierarchy of surgical procedures and stabilization, the position of a pain free wrist through synovectomy, limited wrist arthrodesis, total wrist arthrodesis or wrist arthroplasty, will give rise to substantial improvement in hand function in the majority of patients. There is a group of patients that clearly have quite significant destruction of the wrist or have quite marked secondary degenerative arthrosis that seem to function quite well and therefore there is no absolute requirement or imperative to treat the wrist joint if there is good function. However, any loss of stability, any diminishing of hand function because of unstable or painful wrist should be dealt with appropriately.

4. The thumb: As we move to the hand itself the thumb forms 50% of hand function. This is not always appreciated, but pinch and closure of grasp is a crucially important activity and in general the thumb must be regarded as being the fourth priority in the hierarchy of surgical procedure; whether this be fusion of the thumb or replacement of the joint, transfer tendons. However, there is a requirement to consider the thumb before the index and other fingers. If the thumb is no problem or it has been treated, then one has to look at the next level of surgical hierarchy.

5. The metacarpophalangeal joints: There is no doubt that there is an inter-relationship between the deformity of the wrist and the deformity of the metacarpophalangeal joint. Certainly patients with any ulna deviation beyond 10° to 15° should be regarded as having a permanent deformity, which will worsen with time. There are cases in the literature that do seem to recover not withstanding any surgery just with splints, but the vast majority of deformities in the hand tend to be progressive. All this is seen against a

background of whether the problem actually causes function difficulties or is likely to cause function difficulties in due course. Therefore ulnar deviation, supination of the metacarpophalangeal joints and volar subluxation are deformities to be treated early in their history as they inevitably progress and become much more difficult to treat at a later stage. The results of early interventional procedures although not as dramatic do slow the course of the hand deformities in many patients and the results are very acceptable. The patients maintain their function for much longer, if it is possible to start with a reasonably good hand requiring some modest correction of the deformity as opposed to the patients who have grossly destroyed joints with a subluxation as well, ulna drift, supination, and who require salvage surgery.

6. Extensor tendons: There is an interesting debate as to whether one should do the extensor tendons first, or second, because when one is operating on the wrist the extensor tendons are available and have to be operated on in order to get at the wrist. As a consequence, there is a temptation to do extensor tendon reconstructions at the time of wrist surgery. However, this has a potential disadvantage, if there is very good motion of the metacarpophalangeal joints then placing an outrigger on the forearm and hand takes the pressure off the extensor tendon repairs and allows earlier immobilization with the possibility of good excursion of the tendon repairs minimising adhesion formation. However, if, when at the time of extensor tendon surgery there is a very limited range of motion of the metacarpophalangeal joints (and therefore of tendon excursion), then the ultimate outcome of a tendon repair or tenolysis would be very modest with the formation of significant short adhesions. Thus, without actual excursion of the finger joints, the repair or tenolysis of the extensor mechanism is unlikely to develop a good excursion and therefore in turn there is likely to be only modest improvement in the function. Whereas if there is excellent movement of the metacarpophalangeal joints, one would expect to get a much better result from extensor tenolysis. However, that means replacing the metacarpophalangeal joints if they are stiff *before* one repairs or performs tenolysis on the extensor tendons. That is why extensor tendons come after metacarpophalangeal joints and are sixth on the list of our surgical hierarchy.

   If the tendons are ruptured in patients who are about to undergo metacarpophalangeal joint surgery there is no impediment to the potential motion of the new joints and a lively rubber band extensor splint can always compensate for the extensor tendons.

7. Proximal interphalangeal joints: After the extensor tendons comes problems with the proximal interphalangeal joints and we all recognise that boutonnière deformities tend to be functional even when significant and fixed, "swan-neck" deformities however tend to be very dysfunctional very early in the development of this deformity. Therefore, operations on "swan-neck" deformities tend to take precedence over boutonnière deformities. Fortunately, the majority of treatments for PIP joints involve either joint replacement or joint fusion, or reconstructions of soft tissues to prevent deformity as in the tenodesis of flexor digitorum superficialis across the PIP joints to prevent "swan-neck" deformities.

8. Distal interphalangeal joints: Finally, the distal interphalangeal joints need to be considered in those patients with an arthritis mutilans type of destruction of the hands. Intercalated grafting is a perfectly reasonable option to follow. What is absolutely essential is to recognise that given the uncertain progress of the disease process, there

can be no absolute guarantee that the patient will be able to complete a course of treatment. Given the multiple adverse effects of failure to practise joint protection, the results of surgery can be unpredictable and for the individual the results of surgery may be a disappointment if care has not gone into making sure that the correct procedure is being performed on the right patient at the best time and that the aftercare is capable of managing the patient delivering the best outcome. Therefore, operating on patients with rheumatoid arthritis has to be an event that has a definable potential outcome of which the patient has ownership.

8.2. Special considerations

Any surgery which is planned as a two-stage procedure, where the first stage is made up of a procedure which may not have any material effect on a patient, must be justified even if patients say that they understand that there is not going to be the improvement they hope for. If not a two-stage procedure can be very unrewarding, and this could become disheartening for the patient, particularly if medical emergencies or other events intercede between the first and second stage. Indeed the second stage of operation may never be done. So it is important not to do two-stage procedures unless one can do a definitive procedure such as a metacarpophalangeal joint fusion of the thumb. In addition to doing the first part of another procedure, which may be for example a flexor tendon grafting using a two-stage graft.

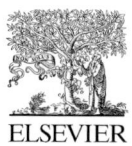

International Congress Series 1295 (2006) 34–42

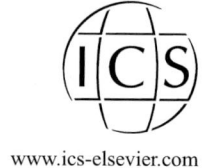

www.ics-elsevier.com

Vascular and neurological considerations in rheumatoid arthritis

Mike Hayton

Consultant Orthopaedic Hand Surgeon, Wrightington Hospital, UK

Abstract. Rheumatoid arthritis is a chronic systemic inflammatory disease characterized by a symmetrical polyarthritis of varying extent, severity and deformity. It is associated with synovitis of joint and tendon sheaths, articular cartilage loss, and punched out erosions of peri-articular bone. Most patients have elevated blood levels of IgM rheumatoid factor. © 2006 Elsevier B.V. All rights reserved.

Keywords: Rheumatoid arthritis; Synovitis of joint and tendon sheath; Articular cartilage loss; IgM rheumatoid factor

1. Presentation

Patients usually present with musculoskeletal complaints. However, they may display systemic and extra-articular features during the course of the disease, but rarely prior to joint disease. These may include anaemia, weight loss, vasculitis, serositis, mononeuritis multiplex, interstitial inflammation in lungs and exocrine salivary and lacrimal glands, as well as nodules in subcutaneous, pulmonary and scleral tissues. The skin and soft tissues need care and attention both pre during and the post-surgical period [1]. Before embarking on any surgical management, the patients should be investigated to exclude co-existing medical morbidity [2].

2. Diagnosis

The American College of Rheumatologists have outlined criteria for the classification of rheumatoid arthritis (Table 1).

E-mail address: Marie.Gillespie@wwl.nhs.uk.

0531-5131/ © 2006 Elsevier B.V. All rights reserved.
doi:10.1016/j.ics.2006.03.042

3. Epidemiology

The prevalence of rheumatoid arthritis is often reported as being 1% of the male and 3% of the adult population female in the United States and western Europe. On average, each general practitioner in the UK, with an average patient list size, has approximately 15 patients with rheumatoid arthritis. A declining trend in the incidence of rheumatoid arthritis amongst females has been observed in recent years.

4. Vascular considerations

4.1. Systemic cardiovascular system

Rheumatoid arthritis is associated with a marked increase in cardiovascular morbidity and mortality. Patients with rheumatoid arthritis are twice as likely to experience a myocardial infarction in the next 8–10 years as healthy age and sex matched controls. Cardiovascular disease often presents at an earlier age and with atypical features.

Myocardial disease due to diffuse fibrosis or granulomatous lesions is recognized in rheumatoid arthritis, although the more frequently recognized association is with coronary artery disease. Rheumatoid arthritis is known to accelerate the development of atherosclerosis. The inflammatory process is associated with adverse effects upon cholesterol and triglycerides. Both low-density lipoprotein (LDL) cholesterol and triglycerides can be adversely affected by disease modifying therapy.

Systemic vasculitis may also involve coronary vessels. Aortic incompetence due to valvular thickening and nodule formation or dilation of the ascending aorta have been described.

4.2. Vasculitis

Vasculitis occurs in rheumatoid patients with seropositive and nodular disease. This may present with severe systemic features classically high temperature and weight loss. Other clinical features include Raynaud's phenomenon, nail-fold and digital infarcts, gangrene, skin ulceration, mononeuritis multiplex, scleromalacia perforans and occlusion of arteries to visceral organs. The occlusion to visceral organs includes coronary, pulmonary, coeliac axis and cerebral vessels. In some patients, vasculitis may present as a skin rash associated with necrotizing polyangiitis of small cutaneous blood vessels.

There are many complex and changing classifications of vasculitis; however, the simplest and easily remembered is that based on the affected vessel size.

Table 1
Mike Hayton FESSH 06

American College of Rheumatology criteria for the classification of rheumatoid arthritis
1. Morning stiffness in and around joints for at least 1 h
2. Soft tissue swelling of three or more joints observed by a physician
3. Swelling (arthritis) of proximal interphalangeal, metacarpophalangeal or wrist joints
4. Symmetrical swelling of joints
5. Subcutaneous rheumatoid nodules
6. Presence of IgM rheumatoid factor in abnormal amounts
7. Radiographic erosions and/or periarticular osteopenia in hand and/or wrist joints

Categorization is based on whether the vessels are large, medium or small. Large vessels would include the aorta and it's major branches as well as the corresponding large venous structures. Medium would refer to vessels that are smaller than the above but still include the four classic components, namely, an intima, a continuous internal elastic lamina, a muscular media and an adventitia. These vessels would be visible as a macroscopic specimen. Small vessels include capillaries, post-capillary venules and arterioles, typically smaller than 500 μm in diameter.

There are two types of pathological lesions involving arterial walls.

The first type is a homogeneous non-inflammatory fibrointimal hyperplasia. This pathological process usually results in progressive vascular occlusion. This lesion is typically observed in the digital vessels of patients with chronic disease and is associated with collateral blood vessel formation. The patient has often a history of intermittent nail-fold infarcts that commonly occur in the colder months.

The second type of lesion has a polyarteritic pathology, is observed in patients with rheumatoid systemic vasculitis and carries a much poorer prognosis. Medium- and small-sized arteries of the limbs, peripheral nerves and organs are involved, but renal vessels are spared. Histopathological examination of involved vessels reveals lymphocytic, histiocytic and inflammatory cell infiltration of the medial and perivascular area, disruption of the internal elastic lamina by fibrinoid necrosis and proliferation of the vessel wall intima with intravascular thrombosis and occlusion.

Scleroderma (systemic sclerosis) is a multisystem disease that involves the skin, gastrointestinal tract, kidneys, lungs and heart and often the hands. The aetiology is unknown but it is more frequent in females than males. Fibrosis affects the skin, mainly in the face and hands. The facial appearances are common and cause difficulty opening the mouth (Fig. 1). Severe finger deformity occurs with marked stiffness and lack of supple hand function.

A common early manifestation is Raynaud's phenomenon, with intermittent vasospasm and reduced digital circulation. During these episodes, vascular changes are dramatic and the digits change colour from white to blue and finally a deep congested red. The resulting digital ischaemia can lead to skin ulcers, fingertip necrosis and eventually autoamputation of the fingers. The acronym CREST has been used to describe the features of systemic sclerosis: calcinosis (Fig. 2), Raynaud's phenomenon (Fig. 3), oesophageal dysfunction, sclerodactyly and telangiectasia (Fig. 4).

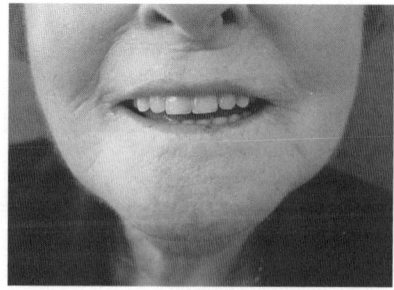

Fig. 1. Typical facies of scleroderma.

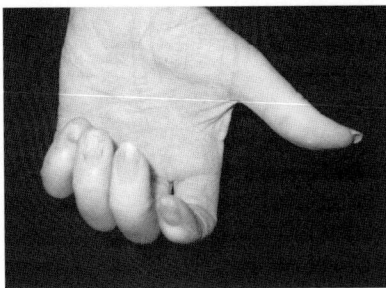

Fig. 2. Calcinoisis: the calcific deposits are noted on the thumb pulp.

Surgical approaches to improve digital circulation have focused on attempts to decrease the sympathetic innervation of the digital vessels [3,4].

5. Neurological considerations

Rheumatoid arthritis may cause both intraneural and extraneural pathological processes that affect the nerves ability to function. The intraneural components will not be discussed in this hand surgery review article and the extraneural compressive pathology will be outlined. However, the intraneural component may be worth remembering if a patient fails to recover from the surgical decompression of an expected compressive neuropathy.

5.1. Compressive neuropathies

Rheumatoid arthritis may cause a variety of compressive neuropathies but the most common are carpal tunnel syndrome, cubital tunnel syndrome and posterior interosseous nerve palsy. The are a number of contributing factors to the onset of a compressive neuropathy. These include synovitis, osteophytes and progressive bony deformity. The increased bulk of pathological synovitis is not easily accommodated in fibrosseous tunnel and cause compression on the nerve, e.g. carpal tunnel syndrome. A progressive bony destruction and resultant deformity may alter normal neural routes and cause traction neuropathies, e.g. cubitus valgus and tardy ulnar nerve palsy.

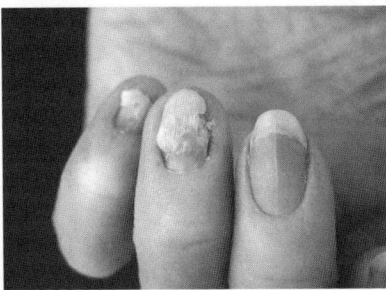

Fig. 3. Raynaud's phenomenon with nail dystrophy.

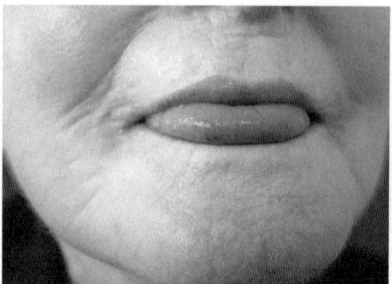

Fig. 4. Telangiectasia.

5.1.1. Carpal tunnel syndrome

Carpal tunnel syndrome is the commonest peripheral compressive neuropathy presents with median nerve symptoms. Patients with rheumatoid arthritis have an increased an increased risk of developing carpal tunnel syndrome [5] Commonly pins and needles in the radial three and a half digits. Nocturnal symptoms are very common and the patient is often woken with painful pins and needles for which they have to shake there hand to gain relief. Nocturnal symptoms may be explained by a number of mechanisms including peripheral pooling of interstitial fluid at night, reduction in muscle-venous pump systems with decreased activity and a sleeping posture with the wrist flexed. However, the onset of such classical symptoms in the chronic rheumatoid patient can be insidious and this history is only elicited upon direct questioning rather than volunteered as in the non-rheumatoid population. Clinical examination may reveal wasting of the wasting of the thenar eminence, positive Tinnel's sign and a positive Phalen's sign. Occasionally, rheumatoid patients have obvious flexor synovitis and present with an obvious dumb bell appearance as the synovitis is bulging on either side of the non-expansile transverse flexor retinaculum (Fig. 5). One would expect significant neural compromise and potential neural scarring but this clinical presentation rarely is ignored by patient and clinician before surgical decompression is performed urgently. Fig. 6 shows the gross synovitis but the longitudinal extrinsic vascular marking suggesting a healthy and recoverable nerve. Indeed, these patients returned to normal sensibility following carpal tunnel release and flexor synovectomy. Occasionally, chronic rheumatoid patients present with simple compressive symptom and signs with no evidence of flexor synovitis. In these cases, I perform a

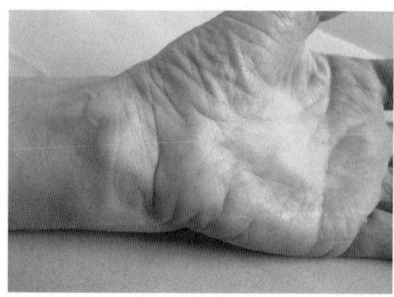

Fig. 5. Dumb-bell flexor synovitis.

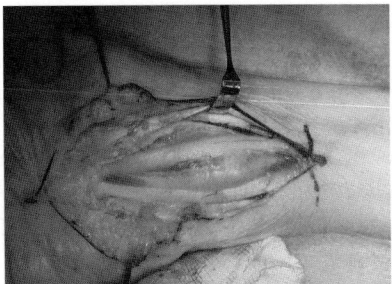

Fig. 6. Flexor synovitis.

standard mini-open carpal tunnel release under local anaesthesia. However, an anaesthetist is always present, in the event a formal flexor synovectomy is required under general anaesthesia. This decision is made depending upon the intraoperative findings inside the carpal tunnel through the mini open technique.

5.1.2. Posterior interosseous nerve palsy

Rheumatoid arthritis may be associated with a compressive neuropathy of the posterior interosseous nerve and has been described by a number of authors [6–11]. The radial nerve exits the upper arm between brachialis and brachioradialis and the divides into the superficial radial nerve and the posterior interosseous nerve. The superficial radial nerve is a purely sensory nerve and continues into the forearm on the under surface of brachioradialis. The other branch, the posterior interosseous nerve, a motor nerve, passes deep and enters the forearm under the arcade of Frohse between the two heads of supinator. Synovitis around the radiocapitellum joint or anterior subluxation of the radial head in rheumatoid arthritis can cause compression of the posterior interosseous nerve and subsequent palsy. The muscles that become paralysed are the finger and thumb extensors. The wrist extensors remain unaffected as the motor innervation from the radial nerve above the elbow and proximal to the bifurcation mentioned above.

The resultant digit extensor lag presents a diagnostic dilemma in the rheumatoid patient. The causes of finger extensor lag include tendon rupture, subluxation of finger extensors into the intermetacarpal gutters or indeed posterior interosseous nerve palsy. However, when caused by posterior interosseous nerve palsy, the onset is usually slow and the patient usually has elbow symptoms and radiographic changes at this site. Tendon rupture is usually a more sudden event and often caused by a specific activity, which may be of trivial nature. Careful clinical examination may also help differentiate between a neuropathy and tendon rupture and there are a number of classic signs that help make the correct diagnosis.

In cases of posterior interosseous nerve palsy, all digits tend to be equally affected, whereas rupture usually is first apparent with the little and ring digits. The tendon rupture may be over a prominent ulnar head, the so-called Caput Ulna syndrome. It is important to note that that the ulnar is in a normal position and the abnormal carpus has subluxed and supinated in a volar direction giving the appearance of a prominent ulnar head.

The tenodesis effect is also very useful. If passive digit extension is present with passive wrist flexion, one can assume that there is an intact muscle tendon system. If the fingers remain flexed after passive wrist flexion, one may assume there is a rupture of the muscle tendon system.

The treatment of a posterior interosseous nerve palsy is usually focussed on reducing the aggravating radiocapitellar synovitis and include corticosteroid injection or arthroscopic synovectomy, open synovectomy in the region of compression.

5.1.3. Cubital tunnel syndrome

The ulnar nerve passes from anterior to posterior through the medial intermuscular septum and travels around the posterior medial aspect of the elbow joint in a groove behind the medial epicondyle. It then passes into the forearm between the two heads of flexor carpi ulnaris. As it passes in this fibro-osseous tunnel, the so-called cubital tunnel, it may become compressed and the site of compression is often called Osbourne's bands. Osbourne described a fibrous band connecting the two heads of flexor carpi ulnaris. The floor of the tunnel consists of the transverse and posterior components of the medial collateral ligament of the elbow joint and the joint capsule. Rheumatoid arthritis may cause a compressive neuropathy of the ulnar nerve in this location as a consequence of synovitis or impinging osteophytes from the humeroulnar joint. Treatment usually involves in situ decompression of the cubital tunnel. In resistant cases or those of cubitus valgus, an anterior transposition of the ulnar nerve may be considered. At this point, one should bear in mind that, in the future, the patient may require total elbow arthroplasty and I therefore prefer the subcutaneous ulnar nerve transposition in these cases. This places the transposed nerve in a more anterior and hence safer position if future bone cutting is required in arthroplasty. In these situations, a submuscularly transposed nerve would be close to the anterior humerus and at significant risk when sawing the distal humerus for implant preparation.

5.2. Neuropathy

Patients with rheumatoid arthritis can also develop a symmetrical, sensory peripheral neuropathy involving the hands and legs in a glove and stocking distribution [12]. This is distinct from the rarer and more severe sensorimotor mononeuritis multiplex mentioned above which is associated with motor paralysis presenting with wrist and foot drop.

5.3. Cervical spine

The destructive rheumatoid process can affect the ligaments, bone and other stabilising structures of the cervical spine and approximately 6% of the rheumatoid population and up to 30% of patients who are admitted to hospital have subluxation of the atlantoaxial joint diagnosed by plain radiography or magnetic resonance imaging. Neurological impairment in patients with rheumatoid arthritis is usually of gradual onset and includes weakness, sensory loss and hyperreflexia.

Presenting symptoms may be localised or referred. The localised complaints may be pathology due to pathology in the apophyseal joints with neck pain and stiffness. Referred pain is usually a consequence of instability and may present with symptoms and signs of radicular nerve root irritation or cord compression. The cervical spine may be asymptomatic, but when severe tends to occur in patients who also suffer from severe generalized disease and advanced disability, and is a recognized cause of quadriplegia and sudden death.

The cervical spine often becomes involved early in the course of rheumatoid arthritis, leading to three different patterns of instability: atlantoaxial subluxation, atlantoaxial impaction and subaxial subluxation.

Atlantoaxial subluxation occurs in approximately 50–80% of cases. It is thought to occur as a result of pannus affecting the synovial joints between the dens and the ring of C1. The pannus erodes the transverse ligament and the dens itself. The atlas (C1) subluxes forward on the axis (C2). Physical examination reveals a decreased range of movement and upper motor neurone signs. Investigations include plain radiographs, patient controlled flexion and extension radiographs, and magnetic resonance imaging.

Cranial settling (basilar invagination) is less common than atlantoaxial subluxation and is a result of cranial migration of the dens between the occiput and the atlas.

The primary goal of treatment is to prevent neurologic deterioration while avoiding potentially dangerous and unnecessary surgery. Magnetic resonance imaging is indicated when neurologic deficit (myelopathy) occurs or when plain radiographs show atlantoaxial subluxation with a posterior atlantodental interval less than or equal to 14 mm, any degree of atlantoaxial impaction, or subaxial stenosis with a canal diameter less than or equal to 14 mm.

Surgery should be considered promptly for any of the following: progressive neurologic deficit, chronic neck pain in the setting of radiographic instability that does not respond to pain medication, any degree of atlantoaxial impaction or cord stenosis, a posterior atlantodental interval less than or equal to 14 mm, atlantoaxial impaction represented by odontoid migration greater than or equal to 5 mm rostral to McGregor's line, sagittal canal diameter less then or equal to 14 mm, or a cervicomedullary angle < 135° [13].

A large multicentre international randomized clinical trial of rheumatoid patients with cervical spine involvement is currently comparing 'early' surgery with conservative treatment, the outcome is awaited [14].

References

[1] J.K. Stanley, Soft tissue surgery in rheumatoid arthritis of the hand, Clin. Orthop. (1999 (Sep.)) 78–90.
[2] S. Schneller, Medical considerations and perioperative care for rheumatoid surgery, Hand Clin. 5 (1989) 115–126.
[3] A.E. Flatt, Digital artery sympathectomy, J. Hand Surg. 5 (1980) 550–556.
[4] N.F. Jones, Ischemia of the hand in systemic disease: the potential role of microsurgical revascularization and digital sympathectomy, Clin. Plast. Surg. 16 (1989) 547–556.
[5] J.M. Geoghegan, et al., Risk factors in carpal tunnel syndrome, J. Hand Surg., Br. 29 (4) (2004 (Aug.)) 315–320.
[6] L.W. Chang, et al., Entrapment neuropathy of the posterior interosseous nerve: a complication of rheumatoid arthritis, Arthritis Rheum. 15 (1972) 350–352.
[7] R.D. Leffert, H.D. Dorfman, Antecubital cysts in rheumatoid arthritis—surgical findings, J. Bone Joint Surg., Am. 54 (1972) 1555–1557.
[8] L. Marmor, J.F. Lawrence, E.L. Dubois, Posterior interosseous nerve palsy due to rheumatoid arthritis, J. Bone Joint Surg., Am. 49 (1967) 381–383.

[9] L.H. Millender, E.A. Nalebuff, D.E. Holdsworth, Posterior interosseous nerve syndrome secondary to rheumatoid synovitis, J. Bone Joint Surg., Am. 55 (1973) 753–757.

[10] S.H. White, J.W. Goodfellow, A. Mowat, Posterior interosseous nerve palsy in rheumatoid arthritis, J. Bone Jt. Surg., Br. 70 (1988) 468–471.

[11] J.G. Westkaemper, S.E. Varitimidis, D.G. Sotereanos, Posterior interosseous nerve palsy in a patient with rheumatoid synovitis of the elbow: a case report and review of the literature, J. Hand Surg. [Am] 24 (1999) 727–731.

[12] C.S. Pallis, J.T. Scott, Peripheral neuropathy in rheumatoid arthritis, BMJ 1 (1965) 1141–1147.

[13] D.H. Kim, A.S. Hilibrand, Rheumatoid arthritis in the cervical spine, J. Am. Acad. Orthop. Surg. 13 (7) (2005 (Nov.)) 463–474 (Review).

[14] J.F. Wolfs, et al., Rationale and design of The Delphi Trial-I(RCT)2: international randomized clinical trial of rheumatoid craniocervical treatment, an intervention-prognostic trial comparing 'early' surgery with conservative treatment, BMC Musculoskelet. Disord. 7 (1) (2006 (Feb. 16)) 14.

International Congress Series 1295 (2006) 43–55

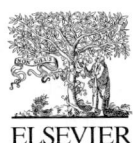

ELSEVIER

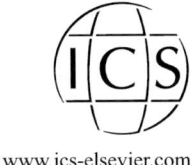

www.ics-elsevier.com

Outcome measures following surgery to the rheumatoid hand

Lynda Gwilliam

Wrightington Hospital Hand and Upper Limb Unit, United Kingdom

Abstract. The measurement of outcomes following surgery to the rheumatoid hand is a clinical priority for hand surgeons and therapists since they guide clinical practice. Traditionally this has followed a biomedical and biomechanical orientation largely because loss of function has been conceptualized on an impairment level. The World Health Organization [World Health Organisation (2001). International Classification of Functioning, Disability and Health (ICF) World Health Organisation] classification of disease has produced a shift in the focus of outcome measures and currently measures that are more meaningful and important to the patient are advocated. © 2006 Published by Elsevier B.V.

Keywords: Rheumatoid hand; Outcome measures; Surgery

1. Introduction

Since the Second World War the treatment of hand injuries and conditions has been emerging as a specialized service distinct from orthopaedic and plastic surgery services in which it has its roots. The need for this specialization came about because of the recognition of the complexities of the functions of the hand [1–3] Hand surgeons and therapists alike are keen to improve and implement the evidence base for their practice. Whilst rheumatoid arthritis is an inflammatory disease, and its principle management is medical, the manifestations in the hand frequently bring it to the attention of the hand surgeon. The traditional stated goals of surgery for the patient with rheumatoid hand disease are (1) to restore function, (2) relieve pain and (3) correct deformity [4].

E-mail address: Lynda.gwilliam@alwpct.nhs.uk.

0531-5131/ © 2006 Published by Elsevier B.V.
doi:10.1016/j.ics.2006.03.065

In the United Kingdom rheumatoid arthritis is a relatively common condition; its prevalence is estimated as 116 per 10,000 women and 44 per 10,000 men [5]. Ninety percent of individuals suffer from involvement of the hands [6]. The meta-carpophalangeal (MCP), proximal phalangeal (PIP) ,and wrist joints are involved earlier and more frequently than any other joints in the body and typically result in significant deformity, disability and distress. Minimizing and delaying the resulting personal, economic and social impairment is the ultimate goal of all health professionals involved in the treatment of this disease [7]. Surgery is one treatment option available to patients, but how effective is it at achieving its stated goals? Are patients satisfied with the results from hand surgery?

The introduction of Clinical Governance [8,9] has placed the ability to demonstrate evidence-based practice as a professional requirement; this means that the continued use of hand surgery in the management of rheumatoid hand disease is more than ever dependant on establishing outcomes for specific surgical interventions. This can be difficult to do since the surgical management of rheumatoid hand disease is still not standardized; many different approaches are proposed, each in a relatively small number of published studies. The low quality and heterogeneity of experimental designs has prevented the definition of universally accepted guidelines for clinical practice [10]. Evaluating the outcome of a single surgical intervention, in an individual with a progressive, systemic disease that affects multiple joints, introduces many variables into the evaluation of outcomes, these need to be recognized and addressed by the tools used for its measurement. This can be illustrated by reference to one particular surgical procedure, silastic replacement of the MCP joints, a procedure that has been well established since the 1960s [11]. The outcomes reported for this procedure, in the literature, have no standardization in their measurement, even for straightforward aspects of outcome such as range of movement and strength, and very few studies use formalized methods of measuring function and patient satisfaction [12]. Such inconsistencies and omissions in reporting the outcome of this procedure have led to different perceptions of its benefits; 75% of hand surgeons but only 35% of rheumatologists feel that MCP joint replacement is a worthwhile procedure [13]. If the surgeons' perspective is adopted, many patients could be missing out on the benefits of surgery, due to lack of referrals from rheumatologists. If the rheumatologists' perspective is adopted, a great deal of money and recourses are being wasted on an ineffective procedure. This underlines the need not only for more accurate measurement of this procedure but of all surgical interventions for the rheumatoid hand.

Within the last decade many tools have been developed that aim to assess symptoms (particularly pain), hand function, impairment, disability and satisfaction in patients with rheumatoid arthritis. These tools range from objective measures of distinct aspects of hand function, such as range of movement, grip strength and pinch power, over more complex functional tests, to different tools for the subjective (patients) assessment of disability and satisfaction. For the majority of clinicians, the major area of interest is not simple improvement of single functional parameters, but more importantly, improvement in quality of life, including function [14].

The World Health Organization considers the impact of disease using a model consisting of the interaction between Bodily Functions, Activities and Participation

(International Classification of Functioning ICF, [15]). This is a more positive expression of their earlier International Classification of Impairments, Disability and Handicap (ICIDH, [16]), but the earlier definition is a convenient way of describing the domains that are included in the instruments for the measurement of musculo-skeletal diseases.

Impairment refers to any loss or abnormality of psychological, physiological or anatomical function.

Disability is any restriction or lack of ability to perform an activity in ways that are considered normal for an individual.

Handicap is the result of impairment or disability that limits the fulfillment of a role that is important to the individual.

Impairment is usually measured by the clinician, whereas disability and handicap are more readily measured via patient-based outcome measures.

Because of the multiplicity of outcome measures available, and the current lack of standardization in their use, the individual clinician must choose which particular tool they will use to measure the outcome of a specific intervention. It is strongly recommended that a well-validated, reliable instrument is chosen, one that is appropriate for the purpose of the study or practice [17]. This process, of selecting an appropriate tool, can be simplified by choosing a tool designed to measure what you want it to measure, i.e., (a) impairment, (b) disability, (c) participation, (d) satisfaction, (e) quality of life and (f) cost-effectiveness. If this method is adopted, then the information gleaned from the outcome measure will be relevant to how the information is to be interpreted and used. For surgery to the rheumatoid hand, the most frequent requirement of outcome measures are (a) to establish the efficacy of a specific procedure, (b) to compare procedures and (c) to measure the effect on the patient.

2. Objective measures of outcome

Traditional outcomes in hand surgery are based on objective measures that measure a distinct aspect of hand function such as grip strength, pinch power and range of movement. They are measured by the clinician and frequently performed preoperatively and repeated as part of the routine postoperative follow-up of patients who have undergone hand surgery.

2.1. Range of movement (ROM)

This is usually and most reliably measured with a goniometer [18,19]. A baseline measurement is made and this is compared with repeat measurements at defined intervals after treatment. This outcome tool allows us to detect any difference in the range or arc of movement obtained through a specific intervention. Often clinicians infer that an increase in ROM following surgery equates to an improvement in functional ability, it does not, it is only a change in the range of movement. In a study that compared the outcome between the Neuflex and Swanson metacarpophalangeal joint replacements [20], the Neuflex implant obtained a statistically significant increase in movement over the Swanson, and although both groups of patients showed a trend towards improved function (as measured by the Sequential Occupational Dexterity Assessment, SODA), there was no significant difference for function in the group with the greatest improvement in ROM and the group with less improvement.

2.2. Strength

Grip strength assessment is frequently used in clinical trials and has shown to be a sensitive indicator of disease [21]. It is usually measured with a dynamometer [22,23] but in the author's opinion, some patients with rheumatoid hand disease have insufficient strength to produce a meaningful reading on the dial of the dynamometer and the use of a sphygmomanometer and other modified blood pressure cuffs that record the lower end of power have been suggested. The use of such instruments does not produce reliable and reproducible results because of the problems associated with calibration and are not recommended by the author.

Again, as with the measurement of range of movement, an improvement in grip strength cannot be taken to infer an improvement in function. The same study that demonstrated no correlation between increases in range of movement and functional improvement [20] also failed to demonstrate any correlation between improvement in strength following metacarophalangeal joint replacements with an improvement in function. Recently, in addition to standard "static" grip strength measurements, tools that measure "dynamic" hand grips have been developed; these are reported to be more sensitive indicators of function than the maximum grip strength measurement [24]. However, such instruments are not readily available in the clinical setting, and although they may be useful for research purposes, their scarcity does not make them useful tools in the routine measurement of outcomes.

2.3. Pinch power

The thumb contributes significantly to the function of the hand and any loss in the ability to pinch between the thumb and the index/middle finger(s) will result in a functional loss. Restoring thumb stability and power is a frequent goal of surgery for the hand surgeon. An ability to measure the effectiveness of any surgical intervention designed to provide this is clearly desirable. In clinical practice, the Preston Pinch Gauge and the B&L Pinch Gauge are widely used for pinch power measurements [25,23]), and in the author's experience, most patients with rheumatoid hand disease have sufficient power to record a measurement on this instrument. For those that cannot, as with the measurement of grip strength, the use of modified blood pressure cuffs, digital pinch meters and customized apparatus have been recommended, but again, because of lack of reliability and standardization with these instruments, the author does not recommend their use.

It is essential that all instruments used to measure single objective functions of the hand are regularly and accurately calibrated; this includes the dynamometer, the pinch and grip gauges, as well as the goniometer. Equally important is that the protocols produced to administer these tests are adhered to, or in their absence, strict protocols are developed for the instrument's use. Without such standardization of measurement, the clinical data produced from these tests cannot be accepted as reliable, nor can we be certain that examiner bias has been eliminated, and we must dismiss the information obtained from this as unreliable and clinically irrelevant [26,25,23].

3. Standardized functional assessment

Clinicians, therapists in particular, are encouraged to routinely use standardized assessments to measure hand function prior to and after treatment. Such assessments are also advocated as useful tools to evaluate the outcome of surgery to the rheumatoid hand. To qualify as a standardized test the instrument must meet certain criteria:

(1) There must be a statement of the purpose of the test.
(2) There should be detailed descriptions of the equipment required to perform the test.
(3) A protocol for administering, scoring and interpreting the test is required.
(4) Statistical evidence of the instruments validity and reliability is essential.
(5) Normative data for the population from which the patients were drawn should be available [27].

The literature over the last 10 years has seen a proliferation of articles describing the development and validation of standardized assessments and outcome measures (Table 1).

These tests provide "objective" data; they combine measurement of grip and pinch strength with functional tasks [28]. They generally focus on tasks that are necessary to perform different Activities of Daily Living (ADL), or they measure complex movements of the hand and upper limb and result in a distinct score. Functional tests facilitate evidence-based practice by allowing the comparison of outcomes between treatments, patients and services, or between time points for the same individual. However, the activities used in these assessments are often artificial and repetitive, their tabulated results, e.g., speed of placing or turning, do not equate to daily life performance or functioning . Generally, these tests measure impairment of the rheumatoid hand. A recent survey of 160 occupational therapists [29] working in hospitals where a consultant rheumatologist was known to be in post revealed that the majority of therapists in these centers do not routinely use standardized functional tests to inform their clinical practice. The reason given by the majority of therapists was that standardized assessments are not helpful with their day to day clinical decision making process, they needed to be

Table 1
Standardized hand assessment instruments

Carroll UEFT(1)
Jebsen Hand Function test
Minnesota Rate of Manipulation test
Nine Hole peg test
Perdue Peg Board
Rancho Los Amigos Test
Smith Hand Function Test
Sequential Occupational Dexterity Assessment
Sollerman Hand Function Test
Hand Function Index (HFI)
Arthritis Hand Function test (AHFT)
Grip Ability Test

These assessments are known to the author, the list is not exhaustive.

performed in addition to a non-standardized assessment, one respondent stated "I don't use them because I've never found one adaptable and flexible enough for people with RA, because deformity doesn't equal dysfunction or even relate to it sometimes" Most of these therapists were using non-standardized assessments to guide their clinical practice; the reasons given for not using standardized assessments were related to (a) the advantages of non-standardized assessments in the clinical setting, (b) access to standardized instruments, (c) issues related to delivery of care, (d) the influence of training courses and (e) those who used both standardized and non-standardized assessments in selected situations [29]. In surveys conducted amongst hand therapists [17] great variation in common practice was also revealed, the standardized hand assessment was not regularly used by hand therapists. Why are standardized assessments not more regularly used in clinical practice? The most likely answer to this is that they actually measure impairment and therapists have long been aware that for the patient, symptoms, especially pain and limitations in ADL are more important than the impairment itself [14] (Table 1).

The existing literature focuses primarily on the development and validation of standardized assessments, and there is a noticeable gap for papers that evaluate the utility of the various instruments in applied clinical contexts [29]. But a few have been reported on and recommended as sensitive and useful outcome tools for the evaluation of the rheumatoid hand when used in conjunction with other outcome measures:

Jebson Hand Function Test [30,31]
The Grip Ability Test [32,33]
SODA (Sequential Occupational Dexterity Assessment) [20].

4. Subjective assessments

In recent years measuring outcomes which are meaningful to patients has been advocated [34,35]. For most patients, pain and limitations in how they live their daily life and interact with others is more important than their functional ability/disability or how that impacts on their daily quality of life. The earliest method of determining the health of a population was to use mortality rates [36]; as mortality rates have fallen in industrialized nations, there has been a movement towards more sophisticated ways of measuring health. This shift was towards measuring quality of life [37]. With the early instruments, quality of life was determined by clinicians, who used various functional indicators, but, by the mid-1970s, instruments began to appear which were completed by patients [38,39]. These early instruments were developed to measure the quality of life in patients suffering from advanced cancer, but gradually, patient-completed instruments found their way into all aspects of health assessment. Scaling techniques, used previously in psychological testing, began to be used, and instruments were developed which claimed to measure subjective aspects of health care alongside the more traditional laboratory tests and objective measures.

The NHS reforms, set out in the NHS Plan [40], have the principles of patient involvement and perspective at its heart. The Modernization Agency, one of the bodies set up to assist with the implementation of the NHS reforms, has as its first guiding principle "to see things through the patient's eyes" [41]. However, the concept of measuring the

Table 2
Self-report questionnaires for the evaluation of outcome

Patient rated wrist evaluation
Wrist outcome instrument
Injured Workers Survey
Upper Extremity Function Scale
Radbound Skills Questionnaire
Alderson McGall hand Function Questionnaire
Brigham Carpal Tunnel Questionnaire
Rheumatoid Hand Function Disability Scale
Algofunctional Index for OA of the hand
Disabilities Arm shoulder and hand (DASH)
Patient Evaluation Measure (PEM)
Michigan Hand Outcomes Questionnaire (MHQ)
ABILHAND
Manual Ability Measure
Cochin Scale
Patient Outcomes of Surgery–Hand/Arm (POS–Hand /Arm)

These measures are known to the author but the list is not exhaustive.

patient's perspective has been advocated in certain fields of medicine for many years prior to the formulation of this policy. Patient-based instruments can and have been used to measure concepts such as quality of life, patient satisfaction, health status and outcomes in different health interventions [42]. Instruments designed to measure the effect of drug treatments on patients suffering from rheumatoid arthritis, e.g., Arthritis Impact Measurement scale (Aims2 [43]), and the Health Assessment Questionnaire [44] have existed for many years, these instruments do explore the effects of drug treatment on the hand and upper limb but in the context of the whole body. It was not until recently, 1996, that patient-completed instruments, specifically designed to measure function of the hand and upper limb and related domains, appeared in the literature (Table 2) Today, standardized, patient-related questionnaires are widely used to assess the patient's view of hand disability in a qualitative way. The move has been away from using the hand disability subscales included in general health assessments or arthritis questionnaires, now specific hand/upper extremity questionnaires for the evaluation of hand disability are preferred. In the author's opinion, there are now three instruments, from a multitude that purport to measure the impact of any hand intervention:

(1) The Disabilities of Arm, Shoulder and Hand Questionnaire (DASH, [45])
(2) The Patient Evaluation Measure (PEM, [46])
(3) The Michigan Hand Outcomes Questionnaire (MHQ, [46])

These three instruments were all designed with outcomes of hand interventions in mind.

4.1. Disabilities of Arm, Shoulder and Hand (DASH)

This is a self-administered questionnaire [35] which includes 30 items relating to functional activities and symptoms in ADL. The patient is asked to attribute a score of 1–5 on all 30 items; there is also an optional section that contains 4 items relating to disability in athletes and musicians. The raw score obtained from the completed questionnaire is translated into a 0–100 scale in which 0 reflects minimum disability and 100 maximum disability. The DASH has been extensively investigated [47] for reliability, repeatability, internal consistency, validity as well as well being accepted clinically. It has been used with a wide variety of shoulder [48], hand [49] elbow [50] and wrist [51] problems. Although the DASH has been used for patients with rheumatoid arthritis, there are currently no published results of its use with rheumatoid hand disease. The DASH is regarded as a good instrument for evaluating patients in a general upper limb practice without regard to diagnosis [52]; however, the author's experience of using this instrument to evaluate the outcome of shoulder surgery, in a population with mixed pathology, is that the DASH is not as sensitive to change for those with a diagnosis of rheumatoid arthritis (and its resulting multiple problems) as it is with other conditions.

It has always been accepted by surgeons that the appearance of the hand is important to patients, but this has been a secondary issue that would not normally be accepted as the prime indicator for surgery [53]. However, this opinion has been questioned, and in two studies into satisfaction with MCP joint replacements, indications have been found that the improvement in appearance may have as much influence on patient satisfaction as improvement in function [54,4]. Since the DASH does not contain any questions on the appearance of the hand, it may not be as sensitive as other outcome tools for rheumatoid hand disease.

4.2. Patient Evaluation Measure (PEM)

This was published as a Hand Health Profile following an Outcomes Conference in 2004 [45]. It comprises three sections;

Section 1 –relates to treatment
Section 2 –"how is your hand now?"
Section 3 –overall assessment.

The middle section has 10 components asking the patient's opinion on several different domains, pain, feeling, movement, use, grip, everyday activities, work and appearance. There are 7 possible responses for each question, the patient is asked to score one of these options. This score is focused on the affected hand. The authors do not claim that it should be administered before and after treatment but suggest that it be given to a patient to complete on their final visit to the hospital or clinic. It is essentially a description of the patient's view of his/her hand at the end of a course of treatments and as such does not allow comparison with their perception of their hand prior to intervention. In the original article, there was no evidence that it had been tried clinically, but subsequently, it has been shown to have good internal consistency, test–retest reliability and its validity has been correlated against scores for clinical measures such as swelling, grip, strength, and wrist movement as well as patient reported pain scores [55]. The testing of the PEM was exclusively on a population of individuals who had scaphoid fractures [55]; there are no published reports of its use for rheumatoid hand disease.

4.3. Michigan Hand Outcomes Questionnaire (MHQ)

This is a hand0specific outcomes instrument capable of measuring outcomes for patients with all types of disorders [46].

The MHQ measures six categories:

Overall Hand Function, one for the right hand and one left
ADL, one right one left and one right and left
Work, one right and one left
Satisfaction, one right one left
Aesthetics, one right and one left
Pain

It is based on the assumption that knowing the function of a specific hand is valuable not only for addressing issues of hand dominance but also for the ability to assess each side separately in bilateral conditions [52]. In this way, it is different from the DASH which measures the disability of an individual rather than a specific hand. The MHQ has been extensively tested and has been shown to have test–retest reliability, construct validity and consistency, it has also been shown to be responsive to changes in the patient's performance, and it includes a section on aesthetics which is believed to influence satisfaction with an intervention [46].

The MHQ has been used in the measurement of outcomes of toe to hand transfers, carpal tunnel release, burns injuries, and hand trauma, as well as being used as a measure of outcome following MCP joint replacement in patients suffering from rheumatoid arthritis. The scores obtained by it correlate well with information gained from patients through semi-structured interviews (unpublished MSc dissertation [56]), and since it also includes a sub-section on aesthetics, of the instruments currently available to evaluate outcomes following surgery for rheumatoid hand disease, this is currently the author's preferred choice.

5. Patient satisfaction

Satisfaction is a concept that is regularly investigated and used as an outcome measure for evaluating treatment. Patient satisfaction is an important and desired element of any health care interaction both for the clinician and the patient. Patient satisfaction is often used by the clinician to judge the success of treatment but is also of interest to administrators and insurance companies. However, the relationship between a clinician's judgment of outcome and patient satisfaction is not always straightforward. Although intuitively, a good clinical outcome should lead to patient satisfaction, outcomes considered "excellent" by clinicians sometimes leave the patient dissatisfied, and those considered "poor" by the clinician leave some patients satisfied. It has long been known that many factors influence satisfaction [60] but Hudak et al. [58] tested a new theory of the factors that influence patient satisfaction with treatment. This theory is based on the premise that satisfaction is linked with embodiment (body-self unity), the more comfortable a person is with all parts of their body the more satisfied they will be (lived body), and the more alien a body part is to them (object body), the more dissatisfied they will be. Hudak proposes that when there is a lack of tension between the self and the problematic body part, there is more satisfaction with treatment outcome regardless of the actual clinical outcome. In keeping with this theory, Hudak suggests clinicians should spend more time exploring individual patients concerns and their reasons for pursuing treatment. The subsequent study that tested this theory [58] concludes that patients concerns can be useful in tailoring or choosing treatment, for example, if the patient's most important reason for having treatment is unlikely to be met, then patients should be appropriately counseled. The study also suggests that these individual concerns could be measured before, and again after treatment, and act as an outcome measure appropriate to that individual patient. This is an attractive theory for the development of an outcome measure, particularly for rheumatoid hand disease where the individual motives for seeking treatment are not always transparent; expectations are variable and satisfaction not always predictable.

6. Patient-specific outcome measures or individualized health status assessment

"Success" in clinical trials is currently measured by scores obtained from objective, functional, or patient administered questionnaires. However, patient's individual concerns may not be addressed or given appropriate emphasis by many of the standard outcome measures. Patient-specific measures are a particular type of measure that allows the patient to state their individual concerns and weigh the relative importance. This forms the baseline assessment (individual concerns and how much they affect/how important they are to the individual), the effect of an intervention is then measured by asking the patient "are you better?" [57]. Although this initially sounds overly simplistic it is a method used every day in the clinical environment and has support from the study conducted by Hudak et al. [59] into patient satisfaction. A patient-specific outcome measure is an attractive proposition for the individual with rheumatoid hand disease and its accompanying multitude of physical, social, economic and psychological concerns and could, in the author's opinion, provide a more sensitive outcome measure for those patients with chronic disease.

7. Conclusion

Great advances have been made in the last 10 years towards more meaningful measures to evaluate the outcome of surgery for the rheumatoid hand. There are still concerns about the assessment tools and methods used to gather information [10,45] and our inability to compare results universally. Standardization of tools and methods between groups is required. Clinicians need to choose reliable outcome tools and ones that are appropriate to what is being investigated; they must be administered according to protocol. The time taken to administer an outcome measure is also an issue for the clinician and the patient and again tools appropriate to the use of an outcome measure should be chosen; if the information gained from them can also assist with treatment planning, then this is a bonus. The outcome movement has refocused attention back to the patient with the development of self-reported questionnaires and is attempting to become more precise with the development of site specific measures. Currently, to obtain a more complete picture of hand ability and the patient's perception of it, it is necessary to use a combination of different discrete hand function assessments. However, when the guiding principle of surgery for the rheumatoid hand is to improve function so that the patient may achieve maximum capacity or autonomy, function needs to be considered in the context of the whole person in his or her environment [15] and the trend towards patient-specific outcomes and increasing patient satisfaction are exiting concepts that may be the future of outcome measures. Perhaps we have come full circle and can return to asking the patient if they are better.

Acknowledgements

I acknowledge the assistance of my colleague Ann Birch, MSC, BA (OU), MCSP, Clinical Specialist Physiotherapist, Wrightington Hospital Hand and Upper Limb Unit, for her invaluable assistance with the preparation of this text.

References

[1] P. Carter, The embryogenis of the speciality of hand surgery: a story of three great Americans — a politician, a general and a duck hunter: the 2002 Richard J Smith Memorial Lecture, J. Hand Surg. 28A (Part: 2) (2002) 185–198.

[2] W.L. Newmeyer III, Sterling Bunnell, MD: the founding father, J. Hand Surg. [Am.] 28 (1) (2003 (Jan)) 161–164.

[3] N.J. Barton, The first 30 years of the British Society for Surgery of the Hand, J. Hand Surg. [Br.] 23 (6) (1998 (Dec)) 711–723, No abstract available.

[4] K. Synnott, H. Mullet, H. Faull, E.P. Kelly, Outcome measures following metacarpophalangeal joint replacement, J. Hand Surg. [Br.] 25 (6) (2000 (Dec)) 601–603.

[5] D. Symmons, G. Turner, R. Webb, P. Asten, E. Barret, M. Lunt, D. Scott, A. Silman, The prevelance of rheumatoid arthritis in the United Kingdom: new estimates for a new century, Rheumatology 41 (2002) 793–800.

[6] E.D. Harris Jr., The clinical features of rheumatoid arthritis, in: W.N. Kelly, E.D. Harris, S. Ruddy, C.D. Sledge (Eds.), Textbook of Rheumatology, 3rd edition, W.B. Saunders, Philadelphia, 1989, pp. 947–948.

[7] M. Altissimi, E. Ciaffoloni, Surgical treatment of the rheumatoid hand, Clin. Exp. Rheumatol. 7 (Suppl. 3) (1989 (Sep–Oct)) S145–S148.

[8] Department of Health, The New NHS: Modern, Dependable: A National Framework for Assessing Performance (White paper), HMSO, London, 1997.

[9] Department of Health, A First Class Service: Quality in the new NHS, DH, London, 1998.

[10] L. Ghattus, F. Mascella, G. Pomponio, Hand surgery in rheumatoid arthritis: state of the art and suggestions for research, Rheumatology 44 (2005) 834–845.

[11] H. Gellman, W. Stetson, R.H. Brumfield, W. Costigan, S.H. Kuschnner, Silastic metacarpophalangeal joint arthroplasty in patients with rheumatoid arthritis, Clin. Orthop. Relat. Res. 7 (342) (1997 (Sep)) 16–21.

[12] K.C. Chung, C.P. Kowalski, H.M. Kim, I.S. Kazmers, Patient outcomes following Swanson silastic metacarpophalangeal joint arthroplasty in the rheumatoid hand: a systematic overview. Rheumatology 27 (6) (submitted for publication (Jun)) 1395–1402.

[13] A.K. Alderman, K.C. Chung, H.M. Kim, D.A. Fox, P.A. Ubel, A. Arbour, Effectiveness of rheumatoid hand surgery: contrasting perceptions of hand surgeons and rheumatologists, J. Hand Surg. [Am.] 28 (1) (2003 (Jan)) 3–11 (discussion 12-3).

[14] G. Pap, F. Angst, D. Herren, H. Schwyzer, B. Simmen, Evaluation of wrist and hand handicap and postoperative outcome in rheumatoid arthritis. Hand Clin. 19 (3) (submitted for publication (Aug)) 471–481.

[15] World Health Organisation, International Classification of Functioning, Disability and Health (ICF), World Health Organisation, 2001.

[16] World Health Organisation, International Classification of Disabilities and Handicaps (ICIDH), World Health Organisation, 1980.
[17] C. Heras-Palou, F.D. Burke, J.J. Dias, R. Bindra, Outcome measurement in hand surgery, Br. J. Hand Ther. 8 (2) (2003) 70–79.
[18] B. Ellis, A. Burton, Joint angle measurement: a comparative study of the reliability of goniometry and wire tracing for the hand, Clin. Rehabil. 11 (4) (1997 (Nov)) 314–320.
[19] B. Ellis, A. Burton, A study to compare the reliability of composite finger flexion with goniometry for measurement of range of motion in the hand, Clin. Rehabil. 16 (5) (2002 (Aug)) 562–570.
[20] R. Delaney, I.A. Trail, D. Nuttall, A comparative study of outcome between the Neuflex and Swanson metacarpophalangeal joint replacements, J. Hand Surg. [Br.] 30 (1) (2005 (Feb)) 3–7.
[21] V.M. Rhind, H.A. Bird, V. Wright, A comparison of clinical assessment of disease activity in rheumatoid arthritis, Br. J. Rheumatol. 27 (1988) 364–371.
[22] D.M. Evans, D.S. Lawton, Assessment of hand function, Clin. Rheum. Dis. 10 (3) (submitted for publication (Dec)) 697–725.
[23] V. Mathiowetz, K. Weber, G. Volland, N. Kashman, Reliability and validity of grip and pinch strength evaluations, J. Hand Surg. [Am.] 9 (2) (1984 (Mar)) 222–226.
[24] D.B. Myers, D.M. Grennan, D.G. Palmer, Hand grip function in patients with rheumatoid arthritis, Arch. Phys. Med. Rehabil. 61 (8) (1980 (Aug)) 369–373.
[25] J.C. MacDermid, J.F. Kramer, M.G. Woodbury, R.M. McFarlane, J.H. Roth, Interrater reliability of pinch and grip strength measurements in patients with cumulative trauma disorders, J. Hand Ther. 7 (1) (1994 (Jan–Mar)) 10–14.
[26] E.E. Fess, Documentation: essential elements of an upper extremity assessment battery, in: J.M. Hunter, E.J. Mackin, A.D. Callahan (Eds.), Rehabilitation of the Hand, Surgery and Therapy, vol. 1, Mosby, St Louis, 1987.
[27] E.E. Fess, A method of checking Jamar dynamometer calibration, J. Hand Ther. (1995 (Oct–Dec)) 28–32.
[28] D.K. Clawson, W.A. Souter, C.J. Carthum, M.L. Hymen, Functional assessment of the rheumatoid hand, Clin. Orthop. Relat. Res. 77 (1971) 203–210, No abstract available.
[29] E.L. Blenkiron, Uptake of standardised hand assessments in rheumatology: why is it so low? Br. J. Occup. Ther. 68 (4) (2005 (April)).
[30] M.C. Kasch, Acute hand injuries, in: L.W. Predetti, B. Zoltan (Eds.), Occupational Therapy: Practice Skills for Physical Dysfunction, CV Mosby, St Louis, 1990.
[31] T.P. Vliet Vlieland, T.P. van der Wijk, I.M. Jolie, A.H. Zwinderman, J.M. Hazes, Determinants of hand function in patients with rheumatoid arthritis, J. Rheumatol. 23 (5) (May 1996) 835–840.
[32] B. Dellhag, A. Bjella, A grip ability test for use in rheumatology practice, J. Rheumatol. 22 (1995) 1559–1565.
[33] B. Dellhag, A. Bjella, A five-year followup of hand function and activities of daily living in rheumatoid arthritis patients, Arthritis Care Res. 12 (1) (1999 (Feb)) 33–41.
[34] P.C. Amadio, Outcome assessment in hand surgery and therapy: an update, J. Hand Ther. 14 (12) (2001) 313–322.
[35] P.L. Hudak, P.C. Amadio, C. Bombardier, Development of an upper extremity outcome measure: the DASH (disabilities of the arm, shoulder and hand) [corrected]. The Upper Extremity Collaborative Group (UECG), Am. J. Ind. Med. 29 (6) (1996 (Jun)) 602–608 (Erratum in: Am J Ind Med 1996 Sep;30(3):372.).
[36] I. MacDowell, C. Newall, Measuring Health—A Guide to Rating Scales and Questionnaires, Second ed., Oxford University Press, New York, 1996.
[37] J.E. Prutkin, 2002. A history of quality of life measurements: Thesis Yale University School of Medicine assessed on line 10/10/2004.
[38] T.J. Priestman, M. Baum, Evaluation of quality of life in patients receiving treatment for advanced breast cancer, Lancet 1 (7965) (1976 (Apr 24)) 899–900.
[39] R. McCorkle, K. Young, Development of a symptom distress scale, Cancer Nurs. 1 (1978 (5 October)) 373–378.
[40] Dept of Health, (2000) NHS Plan. www.doh.gov.uk/nhsplan 20/06/03.
[41] Modernisation Agency, (2003) www.modernnhs.nhs.uk (20/06/03).

[42] A. Garret, L. Schmidt, A. Mackintosh, R. Fitzpatrick, Quality of life measurement: bibliographic study of patients assessed health outcome measures, Br. Med. J. 324 (2002) 1417.

[43] R.F. Meenan, J.H. Mason, A.A. Guccione, L.E. Kazis, AIMS2. The content and properties of a revised and expanded Arthritis Impact Measurement Scales Health Status Questionnaire, Arthritis Rheum. 35 (1) (Jan 1992) 1–10.

[44] J.F. Fries, P.W. Spitz, D.Y. Young, The dimensions of health outcomes: the health assessment questionnaire, disability and pain scales, J. Rheumatol. 9 (5) (1982 (Sep–Oct)) 789–793 (No abstract available).

[45] F.D. Burke, A.C. Macey, Outcomes of hand surgery. British Society for Surgery of the Hand, J. Hand Surg. [Br.] 20 (6) (1995 (Dec)) 841–855.

[46] K.C. Chung, M.S. Pillsbury, M.R. Walters, R.A. Hayward, Reliability and validity testing of the Michigan Hand Outcomes Questionnaire, J. Hand Surg. [Am.] 23 (4) (1998 (Jul)) 575–587.

[47] D.E. Beaton, A.M. Davis, P. Hudak, S. McConnell, The DASH (Disabilities of Arm, Shoulder and Hand) Outcome measure: What do we know now? Br. J. Hand Ther. 6 (Part 4) (2001) 109–117.

[48] K.M. Stute, R.W. Fremerey, J. Zeicher, et al., Outcome analysis following open rotator cuff repair. Early effectiveness validated using four different shoulder assessment scales, Arch. Orthop. Trauma Surg. 120 (2000) 432–436.

[49] K.M. Kuhn, K.D. Dao, A.Y. Shin, Volar A1 pulley approach for fixation of avulsion fractures of the base of the proximal phalanx, J. Hand Surg. [Am.] 26 (4) (Jul 2001) 762–771.

[50] K.A. Hildebrand, S.D. Patterson, W.D. Regan, J.C. MacDermid, G.J. King, Functional outcome of semiconstrained total elbow arthroplasty, J. Bone Jt. Surg., Am. 82-A (10) (Oct 2000) 1379–1386.

[51] M. Sauerbier, M. Trankle, G. Linsner, B. Bickert, G. Germann, Midcarpal arthrodesis with complete scaphoid excision and interposition bone graft in the treatment of advanced carpal collapse (SNAC/SLAC wrist): operative technique and outcome assessment, J. Hand Surg. [Br.] 25 (4) (2000 (Aug)) 341–345.

[52] P.C. Amadio, Outcome assessment in hand surgery and hand therapy: an update, J. Hand Ther. 14 (2) (2001 (Apr–Jun)) 63–67 (No abstract available).

[53] C.A. Goldfarb, P.J. Stern, Metacarpophalangeal joint arthroplasty in rheumatoid arthritis. A long-term assessment, J. Bone Jt. Surg., Am. 85-A (10) (Oct 2003) 1869–1878.

[54] L.A. Mandl, D.H. Galvin, J.P. Bosch, C.C. George, B.P. Simmons, T.S. Axt, A.H. Fossel, J.N. Katz, Metacarpophalangeal arthroplasty in rheumatoid arthritis: what determines satisfaction with surgery? J. Rheumatol. 29 (12) (2002 (Dec)) 2488–2491.

[55] J.J. Dias, B. Bhowel, C.J. Wildin, J.R. Thompson, Assessing the outcome of disorders of the hand. Is the patient evaluation measure reliable, valid, responsive and without bias? J. Bone Jt. Surg., Br. 83 (2) (2001 (Mar)) 235–240.

[56] A. Birch, A validation study of the Michigan Hand Outcomes Questionnaire (MHQ) for the measurement of the outcomes of metacarpophalangeal joint replacement in patients suffering from rheumatoid arthritis. Unpublished MSc dissertation.

[57] J.G. Wright, Evaluating the outcome of treatment. Shouldn't we be asking patients if they are better? J. Clin. Epidemiol. 53 (6) (submitted for publication (Jun)) 549–553.

[58] P. Hudak, S. Hoff-Johnson, C. Bombardier, P.D. McKeever, J. Wright, Testing a new theory of patient satisfaction with treatment outcome, Med. Care 42 (8) (2004 (Aug)) 726–739.

[59] P.L. Hudak, P.D. McKeever, J.G. Wright, Understanding the meaning of satisfaction with treatment outcome, Med. Care 42 (8) (2004 (Aug)) 718–725.

[60] E. Bradbury, The measurement of patient satisfaction. Oral presentation. Hand surgery outcomes meeting, Derby UK, 1993.

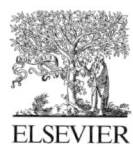

International Congress Series 1295 (2006) 56–62

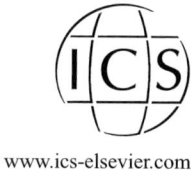

www.ics-elsevier.com

Open vs. arthroscopic synovectomy of the wrist

Lars Adolfsson

Department of Orthopaedics, University Hospital, 581 85 Linköping, Sweden

Abstract. Synovectomy may be considered for the treatment of chronic wrist arthritis. The indications for wrist synovectomy are, however, not clearly defined. Open synovectomy has been reported to provide good pain relief for a relatively long time but can be associated with loss of mobility. Arthroscopic synovectomy seems equally reliable in terms of symptom reduction and no adverse effects have been reported. © 2006 Elsevier B.V. All rights reserved.

Keywords: Synovectomy; Wrist; Open vs. arthroscopic

1. Introduction

A large variety of pathologic conditions, both local and systemic, can cause joint synovitis.

The synovitis may cause pain, swelling and loss of motion, leading to discomfort and dysfunction. Treatment is primarily directed at the underlying cause, but in some instances, these measures are insufficient or not tolerated by the patient and surgical removal of the synovitis may be considered.

The rationale for surgical synovectomy is to remove all actively inflamed synovium in order to reduce the joint effusion and diminish the amount of inflammatory substrate in the joint. It has been demonstrated that the excised synovium is relatively rapidly replaced by a new lining closely resembling a synovial membrane but with differences in permeability and enzymatic contents [12,14,15].

Surgical synovectomy for rheumatoid arthritis (RA) was first described over a hundred years ago but appears to have been only infrequently used until the 1960s. During the following two decades, a number of publications describing synovectomy for RA in most

E-mail address: Lars.Adolfsson@lio.se.

larger joints agreed on good pain relief and improved function after these procedures. The beneficial effects were felt to last for several years. Some even maintained that synovectomy in the early stages of the disease, before irreversible changes in cartilage and bone occurred, could halt the local manifestations of the disease and prevent further joint deterioration [6,10]. This was debated in several publications but three multi-center studies failed to demonstrate any evidence for a preventive effect of the synovectomy [4,5,8]. There now seems to be an agreement that surgical synovectomy in patients with RA can significantly reduce symptoms for several years but the effect is transitory. Furthermore, the findings suggest that the efficacy is similar in all treated joints and that better results are achieved in patients with no or mild radiographic changes at the time of surgery.

Theoretically, any symptomatic, chronic synovitis that has been unsuccessfully treated by conservative methods for a sufficiently long time is amenable to synovectomy, regardless of the underlying disease. The majority of publications on synovectomy deal with rheumatoid arthritis; however, synovectomy has been described as being successful in juvenile chronic arthritis (JCA), systemic lupus erythematosus (SLE), postinfectious monoarthritis, septic arthritis, pigmented villonodular synovitis (PVNS), hemophilia and benign intra-articular tumours.

2. The wrist

2.1. Indications

Several authors have stated that the indications for wrist synovectomy are unclear [9,21]. Feldon et al. emphasize that no studies have demonstrated that synovectomy changes the natural history of the rheumatoid disease [9]. In fact, most studies, as mentioned above, substantiate this. The purpose of a synovectomy of the wrist is not to treat the rheumatoid disease but to provide pain relief and improved function of the affected joint. It is true that there is very little evidence to suggest that synovectomy is the optimum treatment for chronic wrist arthritis but all reports on wrist synovectomy describe significant pain relief, and in most cases improved function, in the short term. There are no reports of synovectomy having any deleterious effect in the long term.

RA remains the main indication for wrist synovectomy. The new generation of more disease-specific drugs has reduced the need for surgical synovectomy during the last decade, but in some patients, this pharmacologic treatment has not been tolerated or is insufficient for the reduction of joint synovitis. As a rule, the patients who are considered for surgery have had persistent synovitis for at least 6 months and have had at least one intra-articular steroid injection.

Other indications that have responded favourably to synovectomy are JCA [3,11], post-infectious monoarthritis and wrist affection in SLE. In these diagnoses, the same criteria for duration and previous steroid injections are usually required.

Arthroscopic synovectomy in septic arthritis that has not responded sufficiently to aspiration, lavage and systemic antibiotic have undergone synovectomy [7,17] success-fully in some cases [3].

Osteoarthritis has also been suggested as an indication for synovectomy. This condition, however, whether primary or post-traumatic, does not primarily affect the synovium and as a consequence synovectomy can only be regarded as an adjunct to treatment of the underlying cause.

Post-traumatic synovitis following a single, or more commonly repetitive, wrist trauma may be an indication for arthroscopic synovectomy. Occasionally, this may be associated with arthrofibrosis which can also be treated [16].

With the possible exception of RA, all the suggested indications are based on anecdotal evidence and some of the described procedures must be regarded as experimental. All reported cases of arthroscopic synovectomy have, however, described good results without adverse effects.

2.2. Open synovectomy

Wrist synovectomy has been described through both dorsal and volar approaches [20,22]. Mobilisation of the extensor or flexor tendons is dependent on the approach, with a large capsular incision to obtain good access. Despite extensive soft tissue releases, access to all parts of the wrist is extremely difficult and a complete synovectomy is

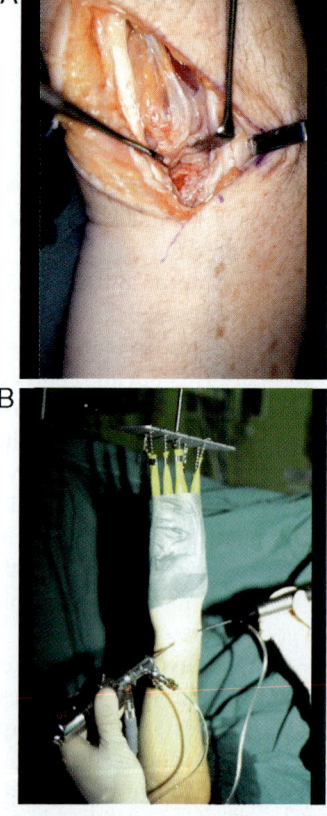

Fig. 1. (A) Open synovectomy does inevitably imply a trauma to the joint and the surrounding soft tissues. Scar formation in the joint capsule and disturbed gliding surfaces may contribute to decreased post-operative range of motion. (B) Arthroscopy is a minimal trauma to joint capsule and soft tissues.

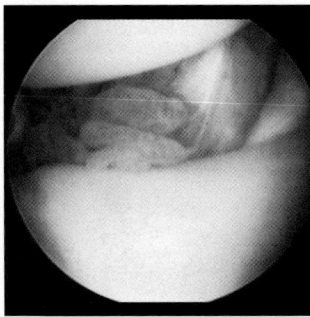

Fig. 2. Post-traumatic synovitis in the radial part of the radio-carpal joint adjacent to the radio-scapho-capitate and long radio-lunate ligaments.

impossible [6,9]. The procedure requires a relatively large surgical trauma to the wrist (Fig. 1A). A meticulous capsular repair is recommended by some in order to prevent subluxation of the joint [9]. Others describe partial excision of the dorsal capsule [23]. Usually four to six weeks post-operative immobilisation in a splint is recommended to protect this capsular repair. Hanff et al. [11], however, allowed active range of motion exercises on the third postoperative day in a series of 20 wrists with JCA.

The benefits of the synovectomy alone is difficult to assess since most publications on open wrist synovectomy often include other procedures. Tenosynovectomy of the extensor or flexor tendons is included in the dorsal or volar approaches as well as resection of osteophytes or excision of the distal ulna. All previous reports seem to agree that good pain relief with preserved grip strength can be expected, but in most cases with a considerable loss of motion. Some studies with long-term follow-up, however, also report progression of radiographic changes and a substantial proportion of patients with late problems requiring additional surgery [11,22,23].

2.3. Arthroscopic synovectomy

Roth and Poehling [19] outlined the possibility of arthroscopic synovectomy of the wrist, and some early clinical results were reported a few years later [1]. The procedure is undertaken using the standard techniques of wrist arthroscopy with a traction device and at least two portals for the radiocarpal joint and two separate portals for the mid-carpal space

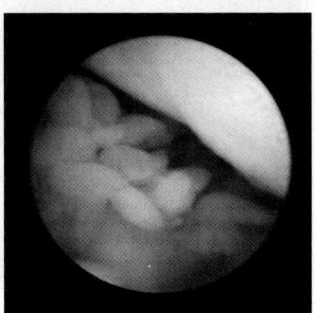

Fig. 3. Chronic synovitis around the ulnar pre-styloid recess in a patient with RA.

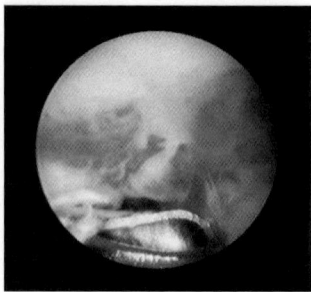

Fig. 4. Active synovitis in a patient with SLE. Shaver below.

(Fig. 1B). The synovitis is predominantly found volar to the scapho-lunate joint (Fig. 2), around the radial styloid process and ulnar around the prestyloid recess (Fig. 3). Normally, the 3–4, 6R, radial mid-carpal and ulnar mid-carpal portals are sufficient to perform a thorough synovectomy [24]. Usually, the mid-carpal space is less affected but the volar and dorso-ulnar parts of the synovium may in particular be involved and sometimes also the scaphotrapeziotrapezoidal (STT) joint in which case a separate STT portal may be necessary. All visibly inflamed synovium is resected down to the capsule using a shaver (Fig. 4). In recent years thermocoagulation has also been advocated [3] (Fig. 5A and B). The operations are done as outpatient procedures and no post-operative immobilisation has been used.

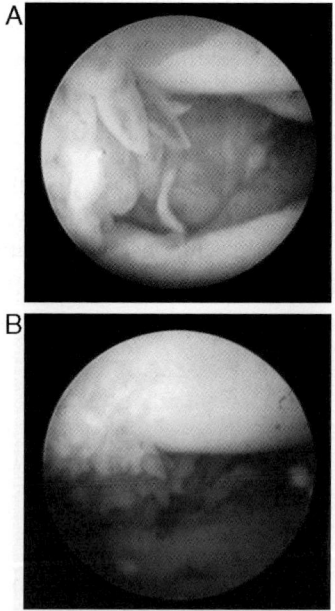

Fig. 5. (A) Synovitis in the radio-carpal joint in a patient with RA. (B) Same area in same patient after synovectomy using thermocoagulation.

Apart from one synovial fistula that required excision four weeks post-operatively, no complications have been reported, although to date few results have been published [3].

No studies have been published with control groups or randomised design but the presented results with intermediate-term follow-up demonstrate good pain relief, with increased range of motion and grip strength [2,18]. The long-term effects remain to be proven.

3. Summary

Both open and arthroscopic synovectomy can reduce symptoms from arthritic joints. In the wrist it appears that in patients with rheumatoid arthritis and mild radiographic changes the effect can last several years. Other forms of arthritic disorders with affection of the wrist, such as early stages of SLE, JCA, postinfectious monoarthritis and septic arthritis may also benefit from synovectomy [3]. Post-traumatic synovitis and arthrofibrosis are other conditions that have also been successfully treated [16]. Studies comparing open and arthroscopic synovectomy of the knee demonstrate that the efficacy regarding reduction of symptoms and improvement of function is similar between the two methods [13]. The only difference being the increased post-operative morbidity, prolonged rehabilitation and risk for joint stiffness after the open procedure [13]. No studies exist that compare open and arthroscopic synovectomy of the wrist. Reports of open synovectomy of the wrist describe good pain relief but marked post-operative stiffness. Arthroscopic synovectomy appears to be at least as effective in reducing pain but also provides better post-operative range of motion and grip strength. There are strong suggestions that patients with wrist dysfunction due to synovitis benefit from synovectomy and that arthroscopic synovectomy is preferable to open synovectomy in the short and possibly also long term.

References

[1] L. Adolfsson, G. Nylander, Arthroscopic synovectomy of the rheumatoid wrist, J. Hand Surg. 18B (1993) 92–96.
[2] L. Adolfsson, M. Frisén, Artrhroscopic synovectomy of the rheumatoid wrist. A 3.8 year follow-up, J. Hand Surg. 22B (6) (1997) 711–713.
[3] L. Adolfsson, Artrhoscopic synovectomy in wrist arthritis, Hand Clin. 21 (2005) 527–530.
[4] Arthritis Foundation Committee on Evaluation of Synovectomy, C. McEwen, Multicenter evaluation of synovectomy in the treatment of rheumatoid arthritis: Report of results at the end of five years, Arthritis Rheumatol. 20 (3) (1977) 765–771.
[5] Arthritis and Rheumatism Council and British Orthopaedic Association, Controlled trial of synovectomy of knee and metacarpophalangeal joints in rheumatoid arthritis, Ann. Rheum. Dis. 35 (1976) 437–442.
[6] W. Aschan, E. Moberg, A long-term study of the effect of early synovectomy in rheumatoid arthritis, Bull. Hosp. Joint Dis. Orthop. Inst. 44 (2) (1984) 106–121.
[7] G.I. Bain, J.H. Roth, The role of arthroscopy in arthritis, Hand Clin. 11 (1995) 51–58.
[8] N. Böhler, et al., Late results of synovectomy of wrist, MP and PIP joints. Multicenter study, Clin. Rheum. 4 (1985) 23–25.
[9] P. Feldon, et al., Rheumatoid arthritis and other connective tissue diseases, in: D.P. Green, R.N. Hotchkiss, W.C. Pederson (Eds.), Green's Operative Hand Surgery, Churchill Livingstone, Philadelphia, 1999, pp. 1651–1739.
[10] D.C. Ferlic, ML. Clayton, Synovectomy of the hand and wrist, Ann. Chir. Gyneacol. 74 (suppl. 198) (1985) 26–30.

[11] G. Hanff, et al., Wrist synovectomy in juvenile chronic arthritis (JCA), Scand. J. Rheumatol. 19 (1990) 280–284.
[12] I. Goldie, M. Wellisch, The presence of nerves in original and regenerated synovial tissue in patients synovectomised for rheumatoid arthritis, Acta Orthop. Scand. 40 (1969) 143–152.
[13] N. Matsui, et al., Arthroscopic versus open synovectomy in the rheumatoid knee, Int. Orthop. 13 (1989) 17–20.
[14] N. Mitchell, N. Shepard, The effect of synovectomy on synovium and cartilage in early rheumatoid arthritis, Clin. Orthop. 889 (1972) 178–196.
[15] T. Myllylä, et al., Consequences of synovectomy of the knee joint: clinical, histopathological and enzymatic changes in 2 components of complement, Ann. Rheum. Dis. 42 (1983) 28–35.
[16] A.L. Osterman, Wrist arthroscopy: operative procedures, in: D.P. Green, R.N. Hotchkiss, W.C. Pederson (Eds.), Green's Operative Hand Surgery, Churchill Livingstone, Philadelphia, 1999, pp. 207–222.
[17] J.S. Parisien, B. Shaffer, Arthroscopic management of pyarthrosis, Clin. Orthop. 275 (1992) 243–247.
[18] M.J. Park, J.H. Ahn, J.S. Kang, Arthroscopic synovectomy of the wrist in rheumatoid arthritis, J. Bone Jt. Surg. 85B (2003) 1011–1015.
[19] J.H. Roth, G.G. Poehling, Arthroscopic'-ectomy' surgery of the wrist, Arthroscopy 6 (1990) 141–147.
[20] L.R. Straub, C.S. Ranawat, The wrist in rheumatoid arthritis. Surgical treatment and results, J. Bone Jt. Surg. 51A (1969) 1–20.
[21] A.L. Terrono, LH. Millender, Synovectomy and tendon reconstruction, in: RH Gelberman (Ed.), The Wrist, 2nd ed., Lippincott Williams Wilkins, Philadelphia, 2002, pp. 365–380.
[22] R.G. Thirupathi, D.C. Ferlic, M.L. Clayton, Dorsal wrist synovectomy in rheumatoid arthritis—a long-term study, J. Hand Surg. 8 (1983) 848–856.
[23] V. Vahvanen, H. Pätiälä, Synovectomy of the wrist in rheumatoid arthritis and related diseases, Arch. Orthop. Trauma Surg. 102 (1984) 230–237.
[24] T.L. Whipple, J.J. Marotta, J.H. Powell, Techniques of wrist arthroscopy, Arthroscopy 2 (1986) 244–252.

International Congress Series 1295 (2006) 63–68

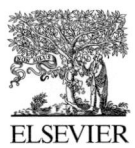

www.ics-elsevier.com

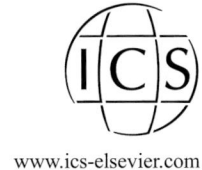

The distal radioulnar joint in rheumatoid arthritis

Luc De Smet

University ZH Orthopedie, hand unit, Weligerveld 1, 3212 Pellenberg, Belgium

Abstract. Rheumatoid arthritis (RA) often–up to 80%–involves the wrist; even up to 95% of the patients after 12 years of disease have signs of wrist arthritis. The distal radioulnar joint (DRUJ) is involvement in 31% of these patients in early rheumatoid arthritis and in 75% in late presentations. It is often the first compartment of the wrist involved. Only a few papers discuss the DRUJ problem in RA separately; usually, the whole wrist complex is discussed or described. The latter are right: it is practically impossible to distinguish the DRUJ problem from other arthritic changes in other compartments of the wrist or to ignore associated tendon involvement. © 2006 Elsevier B.V. All rights reserved.

Keywords: Rheumatoid arthritis; Distal radioulnar joint (DRUJ)

1. Pathogenesis

The DRUJ is a complex joint and phylogenetically relatively young which makes it vulnerable for injury, synovitis, etc. The stability is assured by the TFCC and more particular by the extensor carpi ulnaris (ECU). Supplementary stabilizers are the interosseous membrane and the pronator quadratus.

The pathological events involve the bony architecture with loss of cartilage and osseous erosions, which causes shortening of the bony links. Proliferating synovium also weakens the ligaments. The inflamed synovium causes rupture and/or dislocation of the tendons, more particularly the ECU.

The other extrinsic stabilizers are not strong enough to resist the natural collapse pattern with ventral dislocation of the radius and supination of the carpus; this sequence of events leads to the "caput ulnae syndrome" described by Backdahl in 1963 [1].

E-mail address: Luc.Desmet@uz.kuleuven.ac.be.

doi:10.1016/j.ics.2006.03.026

2. Clinical presentation

The caput ulnae syndrome has previously reported by Backdahl in 1963 [1,3,5] consist in:

(1) weakness of the hand and wrist,
(2) pain on rotation of the forearm,
(3) reduced range of motion of the DRUJ
(4) dorsal prominence of the ulnar head, reducible with painful crepitations, called also the piano key sign,
(5) bulging of the synovial bursae of the ECU and other extensor compartments and
(6) rupture of extensor tendons.

In 1948, Vaughan-Jackson [38] already reported on extensor tendon rupture due to dorsally displaced ulnar head. The loss of supination is often more important than the loss of pronation. Note that, while the ulnar head is prominent, it is in its normal position and it is the (supination and volar subluxation) of the carpus that makes it appear prominent.

3. Radiology

The first radiological signs are minimal sometimes even unapparent. In the first stages, only soft tissue swelling due to synovitis can be seen. Later on the erosions, "the scallop sign" and the diastasis of the bones is obvious. The last stages show severe osteopenia, destruction of the DRUJ and articular dissociation. The "scallop sign" is when the sigmoid notch of the distal radius has an erosive scalloping concavity; this is correlated with rupture of extensor tendons [13].

Besides the specific radiological signs of RA involvement of the DRUJ, it is also important to evaluate the ulnar length, the possibility of loss of the ulnar corner of the distal radial epiphysis, the slope of the distal radial epiphysis, the radioulnar dislocation and the ulnar translation of the carpus.

Evaluation of the radiocarpal involvement is also important in order to propose the most adequate treatment.

4. Treatment

The goals of surgical treatment of the DRUJ are the same as these for other parts of the wrist and hand: reduction of pain, better function, prevention of complication (i.e. tendon ruptures) and cosmetic improvement [3,5,10,19,34]. It is imperative that the treatment is done in collaboration with and under the supervision of the rheumatologist. An important step in the treatment of wrist arthritis is the patient education and the joint economy. Adaptations of work and activities of daily life can cope for a lot of symptoms. Intra-articular steroids can decrease pain in the involved joint and splinting on a permanent base or intermittently can resolve a lot of pain problems.

However, surgical treatment is indicated when conservative measurements have not been successful for 4 to 6 months OR when (extensor) tendon ruptures have occurred. Several options have been reported, most of them in combination(s).

The simple synovectomy of the DRUJ is a possibility but as an isolated procedure no series are available. The ideal indication is DRUJ pain without radiological alterations. It is of course an essential step in combination with other procedures. The same is true for ECU synovectomy with or without relocation.

Bony procedures around the distal ulna can be grouped in three categories (Fig. 1):

- Resection of the ulna: transverse, oblique, hemi or matched, with or without stabilisation [4,7,9,23,29,40]
- Arthrodesis of the DRUJ with proximal pseudarthrosis (Sauvé Kapandji operation) [16,30,32]
- Prosthesis.

The gold standard remains the resection of the distal ulnar head. Although already described in the 19th century, this operation is often called Darrach's procedure. Resections ranging between 1 and 4 cm of the distal ulna have been described. Unanswered questions are about the preservation or not of the styloid, transverse or oblique osteotomy and extra- or subperiostal resection.

The most frequent complication is the instability of the proximal stump. In order to restore stability or the prevent instability, several stabilisation techniques have been reported with free tendon grafts, the ECU, the flexor carpi ulnaris, the joints capsule and the pronator quadratus muscle. None, however, have stood the test of time and there is no evidence that stabilisation of the proximal ulnar stump during the initial operation gives better results. However, a more conservation resection is the preferred method.

The results of Darrach and modified procedures are favorable with 60% to 95% of good results.

Rana and Taylor [28] had in 93% of their 86 patients good pain relief with 87% of them obtaining a full range of motion. O'Donovan and Ruby [24] with a modified technique had 85% of good results. Melone and Taras [22] in their 50 cases had 86% of good outcome with a progression of the ulnar shift in 8% of the wrists. Leslie et al. [20] had also 85% of the patients relieved of ulnar wrist pain. Fraser et al. [12] had better outcomes in 23 rheumatoid wrists compared to 27 posttraumatic wrist, 86 versus 36% of good outcome. Other series reported similar outcomes [17,31,33].

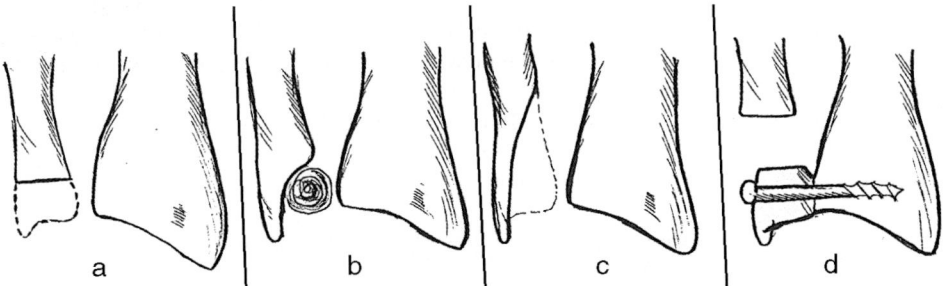

Fig. 1. Different surgical procedures: resection (Darrach) (a), Bowers (b), Watson matched resection (c), Sauvé Kapandji (d).

Alternatives for the Darrach's operations are the matched resection of Watson and the hemiresection of Bowers.

The Bowers operation requires an intact or reparable TFCC [4]. He obtained in 27 patients a favorable outcome. The Watson's procedure is often in combination with radiocarpal fusions; he reported 34 RA patients with a good result in all of them [40].

Silicone capping of the distal ulna has no added value and is abandoned due to the threat of silicone synovitis [35,41].

Another inconvenience of the ulnar resection is the progression of ulnar translation of the carpus. It seems evident that, when the ulnar support of the carpus disappears, further sliding of the carpus is inevitable. Rana and Taylor [28] found it in 10% of the wrists. Posner and Ambrose [26] correlated the ulnar shift with the integrity of the extrinsic ligaments. Cracchiolo and Marmor [6] did not observe further ulnar shift in a series of 42 wrists. There are however several surveys that this ulnar translocation is the consequence of the disease rather than the result of the Darrach [2,11,18,25,27,37]. Thirupathi et al. [36] found ulnar translation in 44% of their series of 38 wrists and found also a linear correlation with the duration of follow-up. Gainor and Schaberg [15] reported that resection of more than 2 cm of the distal ulna could contribute to ulnar shifting of the carpus. Fourastier et al. [11] found an ulnar translation of 2 mm in his survey of 44 wrists; the difference with the unoperated side was minimal (but significant). Instability preoperatively resulted in further progression, but stable wrist remained stable postoperatively [21].

Several predisposing features as an increased radial slope ($>23°$?) and/or destruction of the ulnar corner of the distal radial epiphysis have been mentioned to alert the surgeon and to propose another procedure [25].

The Sauvé Kapandji [30] is in these cases a useful alternative choice. The value of this procedure has been established for post-traumatic as well for rheumatoid disorders of the distal radioulnar joint [8,39]. The ulnar post of the wrist is preserved preventing further ulnar translation of the carpus and stabilizing the ECU tendon, the insertions of the ulnocarpal ligaments and TFCC are maintained and the normal load pattern between carpus and distal forearm is not altered.

Other advantage of this technique that is provides a larger surface so that other (radial) procedures can more easily combined (partial radiocarpal fusion, wrist prosthesis).

Vincent et al. [39] reported in a group of 21 wrists in 17 patients better results with the Sauve Kapandji procedure compared to the Darrach. In patients with a poor bone stock, Fujita et al. [14] (66 wrists in 56 patients) reported a modified technique with a 100% good outcome concerning bony union, pain reduction and increased prosupination, without ulnar translation of the carpus.

The experience with a prosthesis for RA is still limited to case histories.

References

[1] M. Backdahl, The caput ulnae syndrome in rheumatoid arthritis: a study of the morphology, abnormal anatomy and clinical picture, Acta Rheumatol. Scand. 5 (1963) 1–75.
[2] R. Black, J. Boswick, J. Wiedel, Dislocation of the wrist in rheumatoid arthritis. The relationship to distal ulnar resection, Clin. Orthop. 124 (1977) 184–188.
[3] J. Blank, C. Cassidy, The distal radioulnar joint in rheumatoid arthritis, Hand Clin. 12 (1996) 499–513.

[4] W. Bowers, Distal radioulnar joint arthroplasty: the hemiresection interposition technique, J. Hand Surg. 10A (1985) 169–178.

[5] M. Clawson, P. Stern, The distal radioulnar joint complex in rheumatoid arthritis: an overview, Hand Clin. 7 (1991) 373–381.

[6] A. Cracchiolo, L. Marmor, Resection of the distal ulna in rheumatoid arthritis, Arthritis Rheum. 12 (1969) 415–422.

[7] W. Darrach, Anterior dislocation of the ulna, Ann. Surg. 56 (1912) 802–803.

[8] L. De Smet, H. Van Ransbeeck, The Sauvé Kapandji procedure for post-traumatic wrist disorders, Acta Orthop. Belg. 66 (2000) 251–254.

[9] M. Di Benedetto, L. Lubbers, C. Coleman, Long term results of the minimal resection Darrach procedure, J. Hand Surg. 16A (1991) 445–450.

[10] A. Flatt, The Care of the Rheumatoid Hand, Mosby, St. Louis, 1974.

[11] J. Fourastier, F. Langlais, M. Colmar, Le glissement ulnaire du carpe après chirurgie du poignet rhumatoide, Rev. Chir. Orthop. 78 (1992) 176–185.

[12] K. Fraser, et al., Comparative results of resection of the distal ulna in rheumatoid arthritis and post-traumatic conditions, J. Hand Surg. 24B (1999) 667–670.

[13] R. Freiberg, A. Weinstein, The scallop sign and spontaneous rupture of finger extensors in rheumatoid arthritis, Clin. Orthop. 83 (1972) 128.

[14] S. Fujita, et al., Modified Sauve Kapandji procedure for disorders of the distal radioulnar joint in patients with rheumatoid arthritis, J. Bone Jt. Surg. 87A (2005) 134–139.

[15] B. Gainor, J. Schaberg, The rheumatoid wrist after resection of the distal ulna, J. Hand Surg. 10A (1985) 837–844.

[16] D. Goncalves, Correction of disorders of the distal radioulnar joint by pseudarthrosis of the ulna, J. Bone Jt. Surg. 56A (1974) 462–464.

[17] C. Jensen, Synovectomy with resection of the distal ulna in rheumatoid arthritis of the wrist, Acta Orthop. Scand. 54 (1983) 754–759.

[18] R. Leah, G. Rayan, R. Arthur, Longitudinal radiographic analysis of rheumatoid arthritis of the hand and wrist, J. Hand Surg. 28A (2003) 427–434.

[19] S. Lee, M. Hausman, Management of the distal radioulnar joint in rheumatoid arthritis, Hand Clin. 21 (2005) 577–589.

[20] B. Leslie, G. Carlson, L. Ruby, Results of extensor carpi ulnaris tenodesis in the rheumatoid wrist undergoing a distal ulnar resection, J. Hand Surg. 15A (1990) 547–551.

[21] K. Masada, H. Hashimoto, M. Yasuda, Radiographic changes after resection of the distal ulna in patients with rheumatoid arthritis, Scand. J. Plast. Reconstr. Surg. Hand Surg. 36 (2002) 300–304.

[22] C. Melone, J. Taras, Distal ulnar resection, extensor carpi ulnaris tenodesis and dorsal synovectomy for the rheumatoid wrist, Hand Clin. 7 (1991) 335–343.

[23] R. Newman, Excision of the distal ulna in patients with rheumatoid arthritis, J. Bone Jt. Surg. 69B (1987) 203–206.

[24] T. O'Donovan, L. Ruby, The distal radioulnar joint in rheumatoid arthritis, Hand Clin. 5 (1989) 249–256.

[25] M. Pirella-Cruz, K. Firoozbakshsh, M. Monein, Ulnar translation of the carpus in rheumatoid arthritis an analysis of determination methods, J. Hand Surg. 18A (1993) 299–306.

[26] M. Posner, L. Ambrose, Excision of the distal ulna in rheumatoid arthritis, Hand Clin. 7 (1991) 383–390.

[27] Z. Rahimtoola, et al., Radiographic changes after resection of the distal ulna in rheumatoid arthritis, J. Hand Surg. 29B (2004) 148–151.

[28] N. Rana, A. Taylor, Excision of distal end of the ulna in rheumatopid arthritis, J. Bone Jt. Surg. 55B (1973) 96–105.

[29] J. Rasker, et al., Excision of the distal ulna in patients with rheumatoid arthritis, Ann. Rheum. Dis. 3 (1980) 270–274.

[30] L. Sauvé, M. Kapandji, Nouvelle technique de traitement chirurgical des luxations recidivantes isolées de l'extrémité inferieure du cubitus, J. Chir. 47 (1936) 589–594.

[31] M. Schiltenwolf, et al., Results of resection of the head of the ulna, Z. Orthop. Ihre Grenzgeb. 130 (1992) 181–187.

[32] L. Schnieder, J. Imbreglia, Radioulnar joint fusion for distal radioulnar joint instability, Hand Clin. 7 (1991) 391–395.

[33] V. Scara, W. Gohlke, Resection of the head of the ulna in patients with rheumatoid arthritis, Handchir. Mikrochir. Plast. Chir. 32 (2000) 51–57.
[34] W. Souter, Planning treatment in the rheumatoid hand, Hand 11 (1979) 3.
[35] A. Swanson, The ulna head syndrome and its treatment by implant resection arthroplasty, J. Bone Jt. Surg. 54A (1972) 906.
[36] R. Thirupathi, D. Ferlic, M. Clayton, Dorsal wrist synovectomy in rheumatoid arthritis—a long term study, J. Hand Surg. 8A (1983) 848–856.
[37] A. Van Gemert, P. Spauwen, Radiological evaluation of the long-term effects of resection of the distal ulna in rheumatoid arthritis, J. Hand Surg. 19B (1994) 330–333.
[38] O. Vaughan-Jackson, Rupture of extensor tendons by attrition at the inferior radioulnar joint, J. Bone Jt. Surg. 52B (1948) 528–530.
[39] K. Vincent, R. Szabo, J. Agee, The Sauvé Kapandji procedure for reconstructions of the rheumatoid distal radioulnar joint, J. Hand Surg. 18A (1993) 978–983.
[40] K. Watson, J. Ruy, R. Burgess, Matched distal ulnar resection, J. Hand Surg. 11A (1986) 812–817.
[41] R. White, Resection of the distal ulna with and without implant arthroplasty in rheumatoid arthritis, J. Hand Surg. 11 (1986) 514–518.

International Congress Series 1295 (2006) 69–72

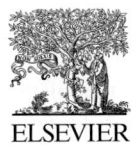

ELSEVIER

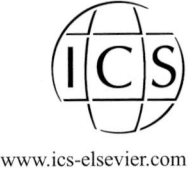

www.ics-elsevier.com

The ulnar head prosthesis
Indications and limitations

Joerg van Schoonhoven *

Klinik fuer Handchirurgie, Salzburger Leite 1, 97616 Bad Neustadt, Germany

Abstract. The ulnar head prosthesis (UHP) has been developed to restore function and stability of the distal radioulnar joint (DRUJ) following failed resection arthroplasties of the DRUJ. Several clinical studies have demonstrated the reliability of the procedure and the favorable results have been maintained over 10 years. Therefore, the method has to be considered not only as a salvage procedure following resection arthroplasties but also as a valuable alternative in the primary treatment of posttraumatic or degenerative arthritis of the DRUJ. Stability of the prosthesis is achieved by means of an ulnar based soft tissue flap. Insufficiency of the soft tissue structures has to be considered a contraindication for the procedure. This may be the case in patients who have had several previous operations on the DRUJ or in a number of patients with rheumatoid arthritis where these stabilizing structures are weak. Therefore, whilst hemiresection arthroplasty of the DRUJ remains the primary treatment option for rheumatoid patients, treatment of secondary instability using the UHP can only be considered if the soft tissues are amenable to reconstruction to allow stabilization of the prosthesis. Other contraindications consist of insufficient bone quality to allow osseous integration of the prosthesis and a previous Essex-Lopresti injury. © 2006 Elsevier B.V. All rights reserved.

Keywords: Ulnar head prosthesis; Distal radioulnar joint; Instability; Rheumatoid arthritis

1. Introduction

Arthritis with destruction of the distal radioulnar joint (DRUJ) is a disabling condition with painful limitation of forearm rotation and loss of grip strength. The destruction of the DRUJ may be a result of posttraumatic conditions like malunited distal radius fractures or chronic posttraumatic instability following injuries to the triangular fibrocartilage complex (TFCC). Other causes include inflammatory diseases (rheumatoid arthritis), tumors (giant cell tumors) or congenital deformities (Madelung).

---

* Tel.: +49 9771662802; fax: +49 9771659204.
E-mail address: hafu@handchirurgie.de.

0531-5131/ © 2006 Elsevier B.V. All rights reserved.
doi:10.1016/j.ics.2006.03.049

Treatment options consist of ulnar head resection [1], hemiresection arthroplasties of the DRUJ [2,3] or the Kapandji-Sauvé procedure [4]. Overall improvement of forearm rotation, grip strength and pain has been reported following each of these procedures. The remaining reduction of grip strength [5,6], the high incidence of painful instability of the distal end of the ulna [7,8] and possible secondary extensor tendon ruptures [9,10] following complete resection of the ulnar head have lead to the advise to limit this procedure only to the treatment of rheumatoid patients [8,11,12]. However, these complications may occur in patients with rheumatoid arthritis as well. The biomechanical and clinical shortcomings of simple ulnar head resection i.e. in patients with rheumatoid arthritis have inspired Bowers to develop the Hemiresection Interposition Technique [2].

The improvement in the clinical situation has been reported to be similar for hemiresection arthroplasties and the Kapandji-Sauvé procedure [13–16]. Nevertheless, as all of these procedures interrupt the bony continuity of the distal ulna stability of the ulna will be compromised. The resulting instability will lead to painful radioulnar impingement in a number of patients following these procedures [17]. Tendon procedures to stabilize the distal ulnar stump have been described but have not found to be reliable in their outcome [18]. Use of a silastic spacer to stabilize the ulnar stump has been proposed but is no longer recommended due to possible silastic induced synovitis and the high failure rate of the spacer material [19,20].

To overcome the painful instability of the distal ulnar stump following resection arthroplasties of the DRUJ and as an alternative operative approach to treat the painfully destroyed DRUJ an ulnar head prosthesis has been developed [21]. From 1992 to 1994 it was designed according to the results of previous radiological and anatomical studies of the distal ulna. The prosthesis is an interchangeable modular system consisting of three stem and three head sizes. Additionally, three stem designs with larger neck length allow accurate length correction of the ulna according to the amount of previous distal ulnar resection. The stem is made of titanium with a titanium coating to allow bony integration. The material of the head is ceramic as it provides the highest biocompatibility. The aim of using the prosthesis is to reconstruct the original biomechanics of the DRUJ by providing the radius with its distal support during forearm rotation and allowing a normal pressure distribution from the hand and wrist onto both forearm bones. Stabilization of the prosthesis is achieved by means of an ulnar based soft tissue flap using the originally stabilizing soft tissue structures consisting of the TFCC, the extensor retinaculum and the joint capsule. Biomechanical investigations have demonstrated the superiority of DRUJ reconstruction using an ulnar head prosthesis compared to ulnar head resection [22]. In several clinical studies use of this prosthesis has been reported to produce reliable and favorable clinical and radiological results [23–25]. This prosthesis has been used since 1995 and the first long-term results will be reported.

2. Discussion

The ulnar head prosthesis was developed to overcome the instability of the distal end of the ulna following resection procedures to the ulnar head or the distal ulna. The reported clinical results have mainly been in patients with posttraumatic or degenerative changes of the DRUJ. There are only single reports in patients with rheumatoid arthritis with favorable results in a short follow up [26].

Patients with rheumatoid arthritis have a lower demand for grip strength and function of the wrist than patients with posttraumatic or primary degenerative changes. This is due to the systematic nature of the disease leading not only to degeneration of the DRUJ but several or all joints of the upper extremity. The primary aim of surgical treatment to the DRUJ in these patients is to reduce the pain and to prohibit extensor tendon ruptures due to the deformed and dorsally dislocated ulnar head. This aim is usually achieved by ulnar head resection although hemiresection arthroplasty should be preferred due to the biomechanical advantages of this procedure. Stabilization of the prosthesis is achieved by realignment of the original soft tissue structures i.e. the TFCC, the extensor retinaculum and the extensor carpi ulnaris tendon. These structures may be insufficient in a number of patients with rheumatoid arthritis and will not allow stabilization of the prosthesis.

Therefore, the primary treatment option in patients with rheumatoid arthritis with painful deformation and degeneration of the DRUJ remains hemiresection interposition arthroplasty of the DRUJ usually combined with other surgical procedures to the wrist joint. However, painful instability of the ulnar stump following this procedure may occur in these patients as well as in posttraumatic patients leading to progressive loss of the remaining function of the hand.

In these rheumatoid patients restoration of stability using the ulnar head prosthesis can be considered if adequate medical treatment is provided and the stabilizing soft tissue structures are amenable for reconstruction during the operation.

Insufficiency of the soft tissue structures has also been found in some patients who have undergone several previous operations on the DRUJ and in these patients as well as in the rheumatoid patients implantation of the prosthesis may have to remain an intraoperative decision.

Other contraindications consist of insufficient bone quality to allow osseous integration of the prosthesis and a previous Essex-Lopresti injury. In two cases the prosthesis has been used to overcome the dorsal instability of the DRUJ following this destabilizing longitudinal injury of the forearm. In both cases recurrent dorsal dislocation of the ulnar head prosthesis occurred. In these patients the stabilizing local soft tissue flap at the DRUJ will not resist the dislocating forces due to the longitudinal instability of the complete forearm.

The preliminary long-term results appear to demonstrate that the previously reported favorable clinical and radiological results are maintained over a period of 10 years. I therefore consider this method no longer only a salvage procedure for failed resection arthroplasties of the DRUJ but a valuable alternative primary procedure to treat the painful posttraumatic or degenerative arthritis of the DRUJ.

References

[1] E.M. Moore, Three cases illustrating luxation of the ulna in connection with Colles' fracture, Med. Rec. (N.Y.) 17 (1880) 305–308.
[2] W.H. Bowers, Distal radioulnar joint arthroplasty: the hemiresection-interposition technique, J. Hand Surg. 10A (1985) 169–178.

[3] H.K. Watson, J. Ryu, R.C. Burgess, Matched distal ulnar resection, J. Hand Surg. 11A (1986) 812–817.

[4] L. Sauvé, M. Kapandji, Nouvelle technique de traitement chirurgical des luxationes récidivantes isolées de l'extrémité inférieure du cubitus, J. Chir. 47 (1936) 589–594.

[5] A. Pachucki, H. Matuschka, F. Russe, Die Ellenköpfchenresektion—Indikation und Behandlungsergebnisse, Handchir. Mikrochir. Plast. Chir. 23 (1991) 318–320.

[6] M. Schiltenwolf, et al., Ergebnisse nach Ellenköpfchenresktion, Z. Orthop. 130 (1992) 181–187.

[7] F.af Ekenstam, O. Engkvist, K. Wadin, Results from resection of the distal end of the ulna after fractures of the lower end of the radius, Scand. J. Plast. Reconstr. Surg. 16 (1982) 77–181.

[8] J. Field, R.J. Malkowski, I.L. Leslie, Poor results of Darrach's procedure after wrist injuries, J. Bone Jt. Surg. 75-B (1993) 53–57.

[9] D.J. Pring, D.J. Williams, Closed rupture of extensor digitorum communis tendon following excision of distal ulna, J. Hand Surg. 11B (1986) 451–452.

[10] W.L. Newmeyer, D.P. Green, Rupture of digital extensor tendons following distal ulnar resection, J. Bone Jt. Surg. 64-A (1982) 178–182.

[11] E.J. Bieber, et al., Failed distal ulna resections, J. Hand Surg. 13A (1988) 193–200.

[12] M.A.C. Craigen, J.K. Stanley, Distal ulnar instability following wrist arthrodesis in men, J. Hand Surg. 20B (1995) 155–158.

[13] D.K. Faithfull, S. Kwa, A review of distal ulnar hemiresection arthroplasty, J. Hand Surg. 17B (1992) 408–410.

[14] A. Minami, et al., Hemiresection-interposition arthroplasty for osteoarthritis of the distal radioulnar joint, Int. Orthop. 19 (1995) 35–39.

[15] A. Minami, et al., The Sauvé-Kapandji procedure for osteoarthritis of the distal radioulnar joint, J. Hand Surg. 20A (1995) 602–608.

[16] P.B. Carter, P.R. Stuart, The Sauve-Kapandji procedure for post-traumatic disorders of the distal radio-ulnar joint, J. Bone Jt. Surg. 82-B (2000) 1013–1018.

[17] M.J. Bell, R.J. Hill, R.Y. McMurtry, Ulnar impingement syndrome. J. Bone Jt. Surg. 67-B (1985) 126–129.

[18] M.S. Petersen, B.D. Adams, Biomechanical evaluation of distal radioulnar reconstructions, J. Hand Surg. 18A (1993) 328–334.

[19] S.D. Sagerman, et al., Silicone rubber distal ulnar replacement arthroplasty, J. Hand Surg. 17B (1992) 689–693.

[20] D. Stanley, T.J. Herbert, The Swanson ulnar head prosthesis for post-traumatic disorders of the distal radioulnar joint, J. Hand Surg. 17B (1992) 682–688.

[21] J. van Schoonhoven, T.J. Herbert, H. Krimmer, Neue Konzepte der Endoprothetik des distalen Radioulnargelenkes, Handchir. Mikrochir. Plast. Chir. 30 (1998) 387–392.

[22] M. Sauerbier, et al., Analysis of dynamic distal radioulnar convergence after ulnar head resection and endoprosthesis implantation, J. Hand Surg. 27A (2002) 425–434.

[23] L. De Smet, T. Peeters, Salvage of failed Sauvé-Kapandji procedure with an ulnar head prosthesis: report of three cases, J. Hand Surg. 28B (2003) 271–273.

[24] W. Grechening, G. Peicha, M. Fellinger, Primary ulnar head prosthesis for the treatment of an irreparable ulnar head fracture dislocation, J. Hand Surg. 26B (2001) 269–271.

[25] J. van Schoonhoven, et al., Salvage of failed resection arthroplasties of the distal radioulnar joint using a new ulnar head prosthesis, J. Hand Surg. 25A (2000) 438–446.

[26] A. Vespasiani, A. Figini, The treatment of the disorders of the distal radio-ulnar joint with ulnar head prosthesis, Riv. Chir. Mano Arto Super. 35 (1998) 1–5.

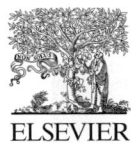

International Congress Series 1295 (2006) 73–82

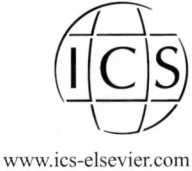

www.ics-elsevier.com

ELSEVIER

Radiolunate arthrodesis in the rheumatoid wrist—FESSH 2006

Nicola Borisch

*DRK-KLINIK, Department of Hand Surgery, Plastic and Reconstructive Surgery,
Lilienmattstr. 5, D 76530 Baden-Baden, Germany*

Abstract. Since first described in 1983, radiolunate arthrodesis has become an asset to rheumatoid wrist surgery. Chamay found spontaneous radiolunate fusion in 13% of wrists and successfully imitated this naturally occurring condition by radiolunate arthrodesis. His concept of stabilizing the rheumatoid wrist has not only increased the treatment options but has also limited the indication for total wrist fusion and for wrist arthroplasty. It has meanwhile been shown that radiolunate arthrodesis can stop ulnar translation and dorsopalmar instability in the rheumatoid wrist even in the long run while maintaining a limited but functional wrist mobility. The loss of wrist motion is on average 38% for extension/flexion and 45% for radial and ulnar deviation. In combination with wrist synovectomy, an important pain reduction is achieved. However, radiolunate arthrodesis cannot stop the progress of the wrist disease nor can it maintain carpal height, as has been shown for synovectomy alone. 10% of patients need a second operation, usually complete wrist fusion, but have no or few symptoms for a postoperative interval of 5 years on average. © 2006 Published by Elsevier B.V.

Keywords: Radiolunate arthrodesis; Rheumatoid wrist surgery

A stable and pain-free wrist is a prerequisite for normal hand function. Since the wrist joint is involved early in rheumatoid disease and progress is rapid, operative treatment is of major importance. It is indicated not only for treatment of established osseous changes with instability, deformation and extensor tendon ruptures but for early treatment of drug resistant synovialitis and monarthritis of the wrist. A considerable number of operative procedures is available: arthroscopic or open synovectomy of the radio- and midcarpal as well as the distal radioulnar joint, possibly with resection of the ulna head, partial arthrodeses, complete arthrodeses and arthroplasty. When deciding for a specific treatment such as radiolunate arthrodesis, type and stage of wrist changes as well as the pathobiomechanic situation have

E-mail address: nicola_borisch@drk-klinikbb.de.

0531-5131/ © 2006 Published by Elsevier B.V.
doi:10.1016/j.ics.2006.03.012

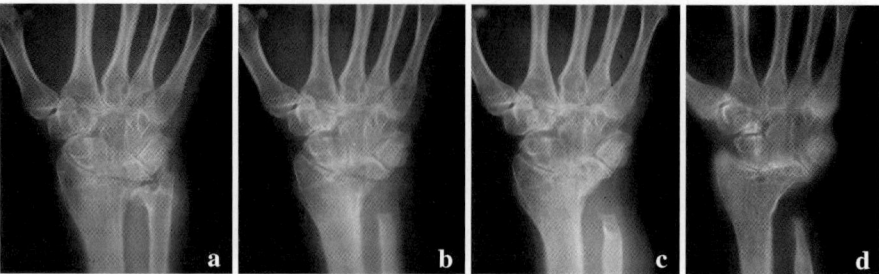

Fig. 1. Right wrist of a 29-year-old patient, radiologic progression over 4 years with spontaneous radiolunate ankylosis. Progressive carpal changes, tendency towards ulnar translation. The ulnar radial articular surface is enlarged in form of a radial shelf (a). After synovectomy and ulnar head resection (b). Progressing radiolunate ankylosis (c). Ulnar translation comes to a halt after radiolunate fusion is complete (d).

to be understood. The individual course of the disease and patient requirements must be taken into account and the basic treatment principles of the rheumatoid wrist have to be considered (Fig. 1a–d).

1. Pathobiomechanics

The proliferating synovitis attacks not only cartilage but also ligaments and invades the subchondral bone at the level of the carpal ligament insertion. Substance and size of carpal

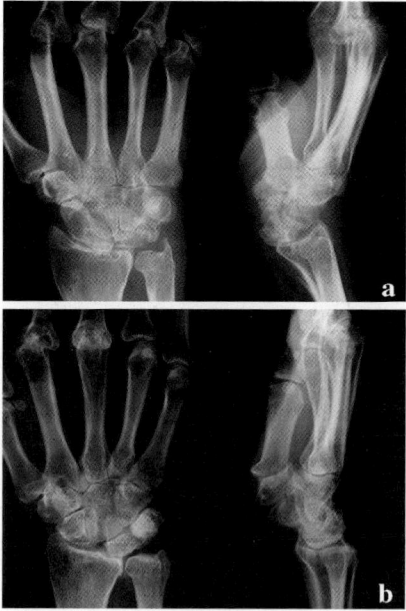

Fig. 2. The two forms of zig-zag deformity of the carpus in the sagittal plane shown in two different wrists (a and b). Dorsal tilt of the lunate with palmar subluxation of the carpus, the capitate compensating is in a subluxed position on the posterior horn of the lunate (a). Palmar tilt of the lunate, the capitate in subluxed position on the anterior horn of the lunate (b).

bones is affected. Radio- and intercarpal ligaments are weakened and subsequently elongate. In this situation, the strong extrinsic tendons of the wrist extensors and flexors which are usually responsible for positioning the hand act on an unstable mechanical system in which the parts are smaller than usual and the ligamentous integrity is no longer present. Thus, carpal height decreases and a malalignment is unavoidable. The proximal carpal row tilts palmarly following its normal direction of motion under load because the straightening motion of the distal carpal row can no longer be transmitted by the elongated palmar ligaments. In compensation, the capitate and the distal carpal row tilt dorsally. This is the zig-zag deformity of the carpus in the sagittal plane. Less often, a dorsal tilt of the proximal carpal row with compensatory flexion of the distal row is seen (Fig. 2a,b). At the

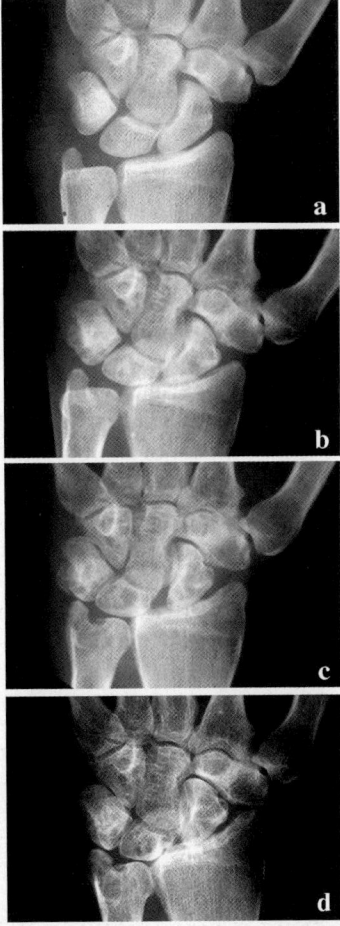

Fig. 3. Left wrist of a 41-year-old patient, radiologic progression over 8 years. Increased soft tissue as sign of synovitis without bony changes (a). Three years later, ulnar translation of the carpus, multiple cysts of the carpus and ulnar head (b). Another year later, increasing scapholunate dissociation (c). After 2 more years, loss of carpal height because the lunate has "slipped" off the radius and the capitate descends between scaphoid and lunate towards the radius (d).

same time or as an isolated event, the carpus can slide ulnarly on the slope of the articular surface of the radius. The distance between radial styloid and scaphoid increases and the proximal articular surface of the lunate, which usually has contact with the radius with two thirds progressively loses this contact (Fig. 3a–d). The ulnar translation of the carpus is mainly induced by the insufficiency of the palmar and dorsal radiocarpal ligaments. It is not the result of the often performed ulnar head resection as has been accepted for a long time.

Synovitis of the functionally unimportant radioscapholunate or Testut's ligament, which originates at the palmar side of the radius between the scaphoid and lunate fossa and inserts into the scapholunate ligament scapholunate dissociation, is most likely induced which can be observed early during wrist disease (Fig. 3c). The result is a palmar tilt of the scaphoid and dorsal tilt of the lunate, which follows the triquetrum in extension. At the same time, the scapholunate dissociation enables the proximalisa-tion of the capitate and thus induces loss of carpal height (Fig. 3d). In addition, synovitis of Testut's ligament often leads to an intraosseous invasion of the palmar radius forming a so-called "Mannerfelt Crypt". When this crypt fractures during pro-gressive disease, the carpus will sink into the radius. A synovitic lesion of the luno-triquetral ligament will induce dorsal tilting of the triquetrum, the lunate following the scaphoid into flexion.

The earliest radiologic signs of synovitic destruction are found at the ulnar head and the ulnar styloid process. Cause is the synovitis of the prestyloid recess, the ulnocarpal and distal radioulnar joints (DRUJ). This induces weakening and destruction of the ulnocarpal ligaments and the TFCC. Thus, the ulnar head gets unstable and a supination deformity of the carpus occurs, clinically manifests as the "caput ulna syndrome". The clinical appearance of a dorsally prominent ulnar head is actually due to an ulnar palmar tilt of the carpus and the hand (Fig. 4). Part of the problem is the loss of the stabilizing function of the ECU-tendon. Synovitis of the DRUJ distents the floor of the ECU tendon sheath. The ECU tendon subluxes palmarly, thus becomes a wrist flexor and supports the supination and palmar subluxation of the carpus even further. With disease progression, erosion of the ulnar head may occur and endanger the extensor digitorum tendons, which can be cut on the sharp edges of the ulnar head on repeated pro- and supination.

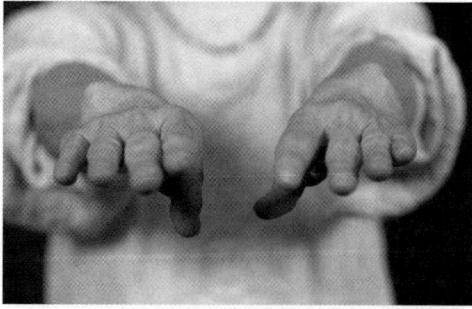

Fig. 4. Typical caput ulna syndrome with (especially in pronation) dorsally prominent ulnar head and ulnopalmar descent/supination of the carpus.

2. Type and stage of wrist disease

When choosing the operative procedure, type and stage of wrist disease have to be considered apart from the pathobiomechanic situation. Local synovitic activity has to be judged correctly. In cases of high activity, synovitis leads to ligamentous destruction before any signs of bony destruction are visible (Fig. 7). This may lead to ulnar translation and/ or dorsopalmar subluxation of the carpus. When the disease progresses in these cases, bone resorption with osteolyses and defects may occur and the disease must then be considered as mutilating. If the local synovitic activity is low, changes are occurring as ankylosis or secondary arthritis.

The surgeon needs to differentiate three stages. The early phase without bony changes and instabilities are the time for preventive synovectomy. The intermediate phase is usually too late for synovectomy alone and too early for reconstructive procedures. Here late synovectomy for pain reduction possibly in combination with a stabilizing procedure such as radiolunate arthrodesis is indicated. In the late stage with gross destruction and instability, only reconstructive procedures such as complete arthrodesis or arthroplasty may be possible. In cases of mutilating disease, early stabilisation of the wrist by total arthrodesis should be performed.

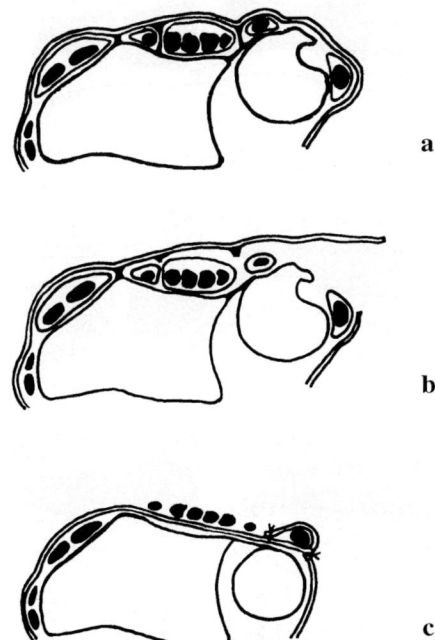

Fig. 5. Schematic drawing of the wrist in an axial view, ulnar is to the right. Preoperative situation with subluxed ulnar head (a). The extensor terndon compartments are opened beginning at the sixth compartment and a radially based retinacular flap is created (b). After synovectomy and ulnar head resection, the tendons of the third to fifth compartments are transpositioned subcutaneously. The ECU tendon is repositioned dorsally and is held in a slip formed by the whole width of the remaining retinacular flap (c).

3. Therapeutic principles

Since proliferating synovitis entertains the destructive process, it is evident that synovectomy has to be part of any chosen operative procedure. Its effectiveness in pain reduction and improvement of function has been shown. In the intermediate and late stages of wrist disease, it is mandatory as well and has to accompany stabilizing or reconstructive procedures.

Extensor tendon synovitis is occurring apart from wrist synovitis, but often needs to be treated at the same time because of the topographic and biomechanic relation to the wrist. This intervention was first described in 1966 by Kessler and Vainio as "dorsal synovectomy of the wrist" and has become known as "dorsal wrist stabilisation" by Straub and Ranawat in 1969. It comprises the synovectomy of the second to sixth extensor compartment, subcutaneous transposition of the tendons of the third to fifth extensor compartment and reconstruction of the 6th extensor tendon compartment with dorsal reposition of the ECU tendon (Fig. 5a–c).

Treatment of the DRUJ which is usually affected together with the radiocarpal joint and the extensor tendons is an integral part of the "dorsal wrist stabilisation". As long as the

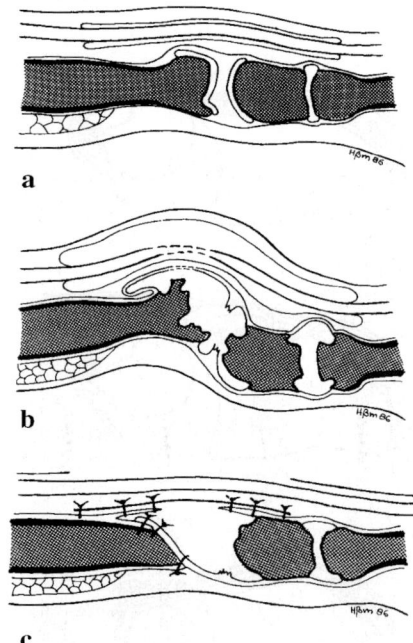

Fig. 6. Schematic drawing of the wrist in the sagittal plane at the level of the ulna. Dorsally, the ulnar head has close contact to the extensor tendons (in the drawing on top). Bony structures are shown dark: on the left the ulna, in the middle the carpus, on the right the metacarpus. Ulnar head and carpus are separated by the TFCC (a). Synovitis between ulnar head and carpus. The TFCC is destroyed. The articular surfaces are invaded. The carpus has subluxed palmarly and the ulnar head dorsally (b). Ligamentous reconstruction to reposition the carpus and the ulna. The palmar capsular flap of the DRUJ is fixed on the dorsum of the ulnar stump. The dorsal defect of the DRUJ is covered by the retinaculum (c).

DRUJ is stable and the ulnar head intact synovectomy of the DRUJ is sufficient. If the articular surface of the ulnar head in this situation is destroyed a hemiresection of the ulnar head may be indicated additionally. Unfortunately, this is seldom the case. As soon as the DRUJ is unstable because of TFCC destruction and the ulnar head is destroyed ulnar head resection is indicated and the distal ulna and the ulnar carpus need to be stabilised by a capsular flap of the palmar DRUJ (Fig. 6a–c).

4. Operative technique

If carpal instability is present in form of ulnar translation or dorsopalmar subluxation, dorsal wrist stabilisation should be accompanied by radiolunate arthrodesis. If in addition the radioscaphoid articular surface is affected for example by a fractured Mannerfelt crypt, then radioscapholunate arthrodesis seems more advantageous.

We have performed radiolunate arthrodesis since 1985 and have used several methods of osteosynthesis: screws, plates, staples and K-wires. Any method is possible. We prefer however the fixation with ortho- and retrograde K-wires because they allow best the reposition of the lunate in the center of the lunate fossa, while plates and screws tend to pull the lunate onto the dorsal rim of the lunate fossa. K-wires are very versatile and enable fixation even in situation with little or poor bonestock, which can be the case in a Larsen grade IV wrist (Fig. 7a,b).

The facing articular surfaces of the lunate and the lunate fossa should be resected maintaining their form. We do not recommend the interposition of bone graft to augment

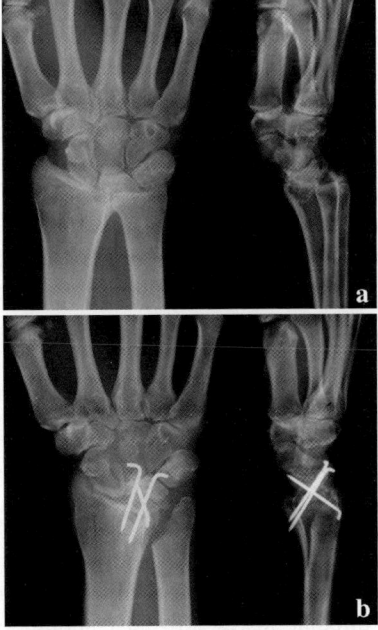

Fig. 7. Right wrist of a 27-year-old patient: pronounced ulnar translation with hardly any bony changes (a). Complete reduction of the carpus after radiolunate arthrodesis, partial resection of the ulnar head (b).

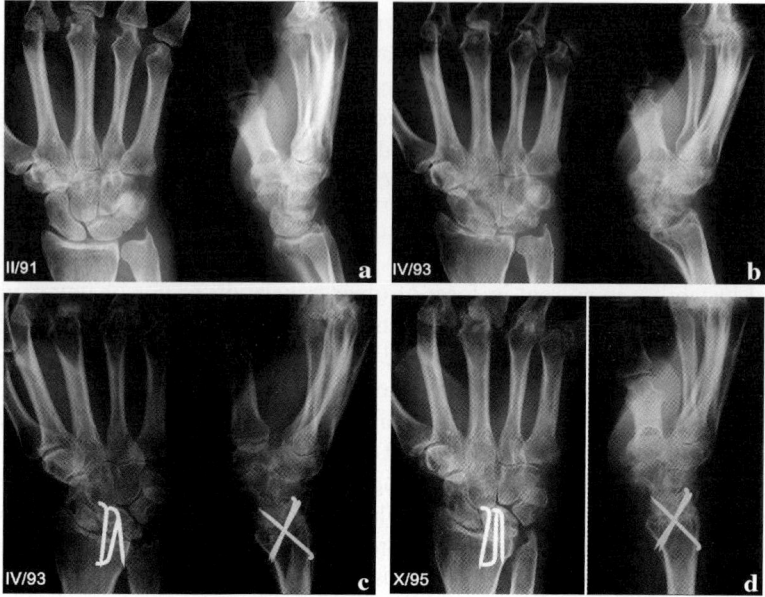

Fig. 8. Wrist of a 45-year-old patient: 2 years preoperatively in normal position (a). Directly preoperatively, there is pronounced ulnar translation and palmar subluxation, Larsen Grade III (b). Postoperatively ulnar translation as well as palmar subluxation are corrected, partial ulnar head resection (c). 2.5 years postoperatively, carpus position and midcarpal joint are unchanged (d).

carpal height. However bone graft–mostly from a resected ulnar head–can be used to fill up subchondral cysts or defects from resection.

The lunate should be fixed in a neutral position in both planes. It should be centred in the lunate fossa in the sagittal plane. The dorsal or palmar tilt of the lunate in case of dorsopalmar subluxation must be corrected (Fig. 8a,b). Reposition of the carpus in the frontal plane should be the aim. However, the carpus should not be forced into an anatomically correct position if this is not easily possible. In cases with fixed carpal collapse, full correction of the ulnar translation may not be possible and it is then preferable to fix the lunate in a "subluxed" position. However, palmar subluxation of the carpus should always be corrected.

5. Postoperative treatment

The active mobilisation of the fingers should begin immediately postoperative. If wound healing is without problems and the arthodesis is stable enough careful active wrist mobilisation out of the cast can be started. However, for the first 3 weeks, this should be limited for wrist flexion. No wrist extension should be exercised before the end of 3 weeks. This should be applied after any dorsal wrist stabilisation, not only after radiolunate arthrodesis. If the osteosynthesis is not stable enough to allow early wrist mobilisation, a circular lower arm cast should be applied for 6 weeks and wrist mobilisation started after the 6-week radiologic assessment. If accompanying surgery of the DRUJ has been performed and the stabilisation of the distal ulnar stump is not solid enough pro- and supination should also be limited for 6 weeks in an appropriate cast.

6. Indication for radiolunate arthrodesis

The indication for radiolunate arthrodesis is principally given when ulnar translation and/or palmar subluxation of the carpus is present on preoperative X-rays. In uncertain cases, it is useful to analyse a sequence of wrist X-rays of the same patient. Progressive ulnar translation may only then become evident. If no such sequence of X-rays is present carpal stability should be tested intraoperatively. Even after dorsal access to the radicarpal joint for synovectomy passive translation of the carpus will show abnormal mobility or laxity of the palmar radiocarpal ligaments. In no case should the indication solely be based on the radiographic measurement of a carpal translation index.

The midcarpal joint ideally should be intact but this is not an absolute prerequisite. Indication should not be limited to Larsen Grades II and III as has been proposed by most authors. The radiologic results are indeed best in wrists with Larsen Grade II but clinical results are also very good in Grade IV wrists. We therefore do not consider advanced rheumatoid disease a contraindication for the procedure (Fig. 9). Here radiolunate arthrodesis is an interesting differential indication for complete wrist fusion or alloarthroplasty. However, cases with mutilating disease will not be sufficiently stabilised and are better treated by a total wrist fusion.

Radiolunate arthrodesis does not invariably lead to secondary arthrosis of the midcarpal joint as has been generally suspected. One third of midcarpal joints remain completely unchanged after radiolunate arthrodesis. However, even if further arthritic destruction or secondary arthrosis occurs, the carpus shows an amazing capacity of adaptation, which can be relied on when indicating the procedure. The carpus remains "hooked" on the lunate and a new intracarpal joint line develops or the midcarpal joint reestablishes itself.

In cases with fixed carpal collapse, usually wrists with advanced disease, one should not attempt to reposition the lunate anatomically or to restore carpal height. This may lead to increased pressure in the midcarpal joint and in our experience may cause midcarpal subluxation or rotation or may precipitate secondary arthrosis. In these cases, we now

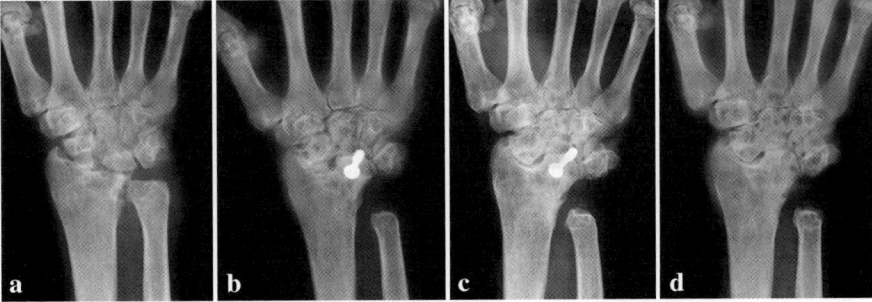

Fig. 9. X-rays of a 45-year-old patient: preoperatively active arthritis, Larsen Grade III/ IV, the midcarpal joint space is hardly visible, possible necrosis of the capitate head (a). One year after radiolunate arthrodesis, the midcarpal joint space is visible again (b). The midcarpal joint space rebuilds itself (c). 10 years postoperatively, a new perilunate joint space is visible. The wrist has pain-free motion of 28°–0°–16° for extension/flexion (d).

perform the radiolunate arthrodesis in the subluxed position. This still seems preferable to a total radiocarpal arthrodesis with its disabling consequences or a prosthetic arthroplasty with its uncertain long-term results.

However, the indication must always been seen in the possible context of a polyarticular disease of the upper extremity, of bilateral wrist disease and the general situation, limitations and needs of the individual patient.

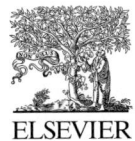

International Congress Series 1295 (2006) 83–93

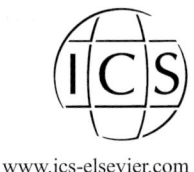

www.ics-elsevier.com

Total wrist arthroplasty for rheumatoid arthritis

Brian D. Adams*

University of Iowa Hospitals and Clinics, Department of Orthopaedics and Rehabilitation, 200 Hawkins Dr., Iowa City, IA 52242-1008, United States

Abstract. Total wrist arthroplasty cannot duplicate the complex mechanics of the normal wrist which involves multiple articulations among the radius, ulna, and carpal bones. However, newer implant designs attempt to simplify this intricate system while producing a stable, pain-free joint with a functional range of motion. A motion-preserving alternative to wrist arthrodesis is of particular importance when treating patients who are debilitated by arthritis afflicting multiple joints. Total wrist arthroplasty enhances the performance of daily activities and is preferred to arthrodesis by rheumatoid patients [M.J. Goodman, et al., Arthroplasty of the rheumatoid wrist with silicone rubber: an early evaluation. J. Hand Surg. [Am.] 5 (2) (1980) 114–121; A.J. Vicar, R.I. Burton, Surgical management of the rheumatoid wrist-fusion or arthroplasty. J. Hand Surg. [Am.] 11 (6) (1986) 790–797]. Other patients may also choose arthroplasty over arthrodesis to better maintain their ability to perform vocational and avocational activities. Regardless of the need or desire for arthroplasty, the patient must accept and commit to a lifetime of restricted activities imposed by an artificial wrist. The patient must also recognize the risk of implant failure with the consequent need for revision surgery. This article discusses the history, technique, and outcomes of total wrist arthroplasty with emphases on new implant designs and strategies to minimize risks and manage complications. © 2006 Elsevier B.V. All rights reserved.

Keywords: Total wrist arthroplasty; Wrist arthritis; Rheumatoid wrist; Wrist replacement

1. Historical perspective

The Swanson implant was the first wrist implant having wide U.S. commercial distribution. The implant is made of silicone that acts as a flexible spacer whereby wrist motion results from a combination of implant flexibility and pistoning within the medullary canals of the radius and metacarpal [3]. Early results were generally gratifying

---

* Tel.: +1 319 353 6222; fax: +1 319 353 6754.
E-mail address: brian-d-adams@uiowa.edu.

0531-5131/ © 2006 Elsevier B.V. All rights reserved.
doi:10.1016/j.ics.2006.03.031

with good pain relief and an acceptable range of motion, however restoration of wrist height and hand balance were unpredictable. Longer follow-up revealed subsidence within the bone and a high incidence of implant breakage, reaching 52% at 72 months [1,4–6]. Silicone synovitis became an important issue later, though the incidence was lower than with carpal implants [7].

Early articulated total wrist prostheses were semi-constrained and incorporated bearings with small surface areas. These designs were intended to maximize flexion and extension, however problems with instability and imbalance were common [4,8]. Various stem designs for fixation in the radius and carpus were tried. Carpal components were typically fixed in the metacarpal canals with cement. A high incidence of loosening marked by metacarpal erosion and implant penetration occurred. Periprosthetic bone resorption of the distal radius was also common [9]. Early design changes focused on reducing wrist imbalance and distal component loosening by more accurately reproducing normal wrist kinematics through changes in the articulation's position and constraint. The revised Meuli (Sulzer Orthopaedics Ltd, Winterthur, Switzerland), Trispherical (Osteonics, Allendale, NJ) and revised Voltz (Howmedica, Rutherford, NJ) each provided satisfactory early clinical results but further follow up revealed continued problems with imbalance, subsidence, and loosening [9–15]. The Biax (DePuy, Warsaw, IN) introduced an ellipsoidal-shaped articulation that demonstrated improved wrist balance. Results were good in the majority of patients but loosening remained a substantial problem. Eight of eleven failures in one series of 58 Biax implants were secondary to distal component loosening and subsidence, which often resulted in penetration through the dorsum of the third metacarpal. A study investigating the use of the Biax prosthesis incorporating a longer metacarpal stem for primary total wrist arthroplasty in 17 patients with radiographic evidence of poor bone quality showed more favorable survivorship with no failures at average 6-year follow-up [16]. The anatomic physiologic (APH) implant (Implant-Service Vertreibs-GmbH, Hamburg, Germany) was designed with a titanium articulation [15]. Mid-term follow-up revealed a very high failure rate. Of 40 patients at an average 52-month follow-up, 39 underwent revision to an arthrodesis. Isolated loosening of the carpal component was the most common mode of failure. Titanium wear debris was found in the soft tissues of all revision cases and was thought to be the primary contributing factor to early periprosthetic bone resorption [17]. The Universal prosthesis (Kineticos Medical Inc [KMI], Carlsbad, CA) combined the concepts of containing fixation within the carpus, augmenting distal component fixation using screws, and performing an intercarpal fusion [18]. The design and method proved to be more durable but the bearing shape was prone to instability.

The overall experience with different designs during the last three and half decades strongly indicates there are specific criteria to optimize the clinical results [19]. Distal component fixation should be primarily within the carpus rather than relying on the metacarpal canals. It should be combined with a solid intercarpal fusion to provide broad support for the component. Using screws to augment initial fixation has been shown to be effective [20]. The radial component should be shaped to minimize bone resection which preserves the joint capsule thereby enhancing prosthetic stability and wrist balance. In patients with adequate bone quality, fixation by osteointegration rather than cement would seem to be a better choice for both components to improve durability and reduce bone

a   b

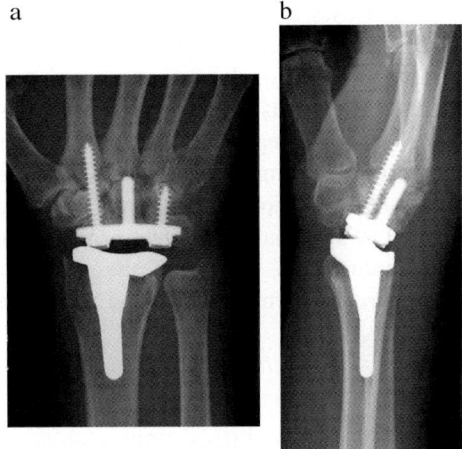

Fig. 1. (a,b) Universal 2 implant, with preservation of the ulnar head and distal radioulnar joint.

destruction if revision is necessary. The articulation should be broad, generally ellipsoidal in shape, and semi-constrained [19]. It should also resist imbalance and instability and yet provide a functional range of motion that can be achieved early with minimal formal rehabilitation. Finally, there should be the option to preserve the ulnar head and distal radioulnar joint. These criteria were incorporated in the design of the Universal 2 implant (Kineticos Medical Inc [KMI], Carlsbad, CA) (Fig. 1a,b) and other implants that are under development.

2. Patient selection

The objective of total wrist arthroplasty is to maintain or improve wrist motion while relieving pain and correcting deformity. Patients who have the greatest need for maintaining wrist motion are those afflicted by arthritis involving multiple upper extremity joints and those with specific needs or desires to maintain motion. Patients with rheumatoid arthritis who have bilateral wrist arthritis as well as elbow and shoulder involvement are particularly good candidates. Individuals who have had a wrist fusion on one side and total wrist arthroplasty on the other prefer the arthroplasty [2,9]. Basic activities of daily living such as perineal care, fastening buttons, combing hair, and writing are made easier if some wrist motion, particularly flexion, is preserved [21,22]. Patients with post-traumatic or degenerative osteoarthritis may also be candidates for total wrist arthroplasty. Because these patients typically have good bone quality, muscle strength, and wrist alignment the result can be excellent. However, this type of patient should be choosing arthroplasty to maintain dexterity for activities of daily living and specific low demand activities rather than to increase their activity level, and they must be willing to accept permanent activity restrictions.

Rheumatoid patients with highly active synovitis that is producing severe bony erosions or joint hyperlaxity have a higher risk for implant instability and loosening. These patients are better treated by arthrodesis. Regular use of the upper extremities for support during ambulation or transfers is a contraindication; however intermittent use of crutches or a cane is acceptable if the patient uses a wrist splint. Absolute contraindications for total wrist arthroplasty include a minimally functional hand, recent infection, and lack of wrist extension power either due to ruptures of the extensor carpi radialis brevis and longus tendons or a radial nerve palsy. There must be adequate bone stock and quality to support the implant, especially the carpal component. Implantation in patients with severe ostoeopenia, bone erosion, or joint deformity is more challenging and the implant fixation is less durable. Previous surgical fusion or proximal row carpectomy are relative contraindications. These patients must have adequate carpus remaining and intact wrist extensors to convert to an arthroplasty. Although the procedure is more technically challenging after these procedures, the implantation and functional outcome can be very good.

3. Preoperative planning

Patients with rheumatoid arthritis should have a full preoperative evaluation including the cervical spine. Total hip or knee replacement should be performed prior to wrist arthroplasty to avoid weight bearing on the wrist prosthesis during rehabilitation. Wrist replacement may be done before or after shoulder or elbow surgery but should usually be performed prior to procedures on the digits in order to optimize joint alignment and tendon tension in the hand. To reduce the risk of infection and wound healing problems, temporarily stopping medications such as methotrexate and other immune modulating medications should be considered after consulting with the patient's rheumatologist. The risk of bleeding complications is reduced by decreasing or eliminating non-steroidal anti-inflammatory agents for at least 10 days prior to and 5 days after surgery.

Radiographic assessment of bone quality, erosions, carpal collapse, carpal ulnar translation, volar subluxation, and the condition of the distal radioulnar joint will prepare the surgeon to optimize the technique and avoid potential difficulties. Implant size and alignment within the bones can be predicted using radiographic templates.

3.1. Operative technique

Although the technique for implantation of the Universal 2 Total Wrist Implant System (KMI, San Diego, California) will be described, there are many similarities to other systems currently in use.

4. Templating

In the PA view the radial component should not extend beyond the edge of the radial styloid. The carpal component should not extend more than 2 mm over the margins of the carpus at the level of the osteotomy. In general the smaller implant should be selected when deciding between two sizes. The optimum size is typically found when the carpal stem is aligned with center of capitate and the ulnar screw enters the proximal pole of the hamate.

5. Operative procedure

Preoperative antibiotic is administered. An arm tourniquet is used. A wide strip of adhesive drape is applied to the dorsum of the wrist and hand to help protect the skin. A dorsal longitudinal incision is made over the wrist in line with the third metacarpal. The skin and subcutaneous tissue are elevated together to reduce the risk of skin necrosis and to protect the sensory branches of the radial and ulnar nerves. The sixth dorsal extensor (ECU) compartment is opened along its volar margin. The entire retinaculum is elevated radially to the septum between the first and second extensor compartments. An extensor tenosynovectomy is performed if needed. The integrity of the extensor carpi radialis brevis and longus are confirmed. The dorsal wrist capsule is raised in continuity with the dorsal distal radioulnar joint (DRUJ) capsule and the periosteum over the distal 1 cm of the radius as a distally based rectangular flap (Fig. 2). If the distal ulna is to be preserved, the interval between the capsule and the dorsal, distal radioulnar ligament is carefully divided and the capsule is raised distally in order to preserve the horizontal components of the triangular fibrocartilage complex. The sides of the flap are made in the floors of the first and sixth extensor compartments. The brachioradialis and first extensor compartment are elevated subperiosteally from the distal portion of the radial styloid. The wrist is fully flexed to expose the joint. Synovectomies of the radiocarpal and distal radioulnar joints are performed when needed. If the distal radioulnar joint is arthritic, the distal ulna is resected through its neck or rounded to create a hemiresection arthroplasty of the DRUJ.

5.1. Radial component

Preparation for radial component implantation begins by inserting an alignment rod into the canal of the radius. To insert the rod, a hole is made with an awl about 5 mm volar to the dorsal lip of the distal radius, just radial to Lister's tubercle. Fluoroscopy confirms central placement of the rod in the canal (Fig. 3). The radial guide bar and cutting block are mounted on the rod and positioned to remove only the articular surface. Lister's tubercle may need to be removed for full seating of the block. After temporary fixation pins are inserted through the block, the alignment rod is removed, and the osteotomy is performed with an oscillating saw (Fig. 4). If the DRUJ is to be preserved, the cut is stopped approximately 5 mm short of the sigmoid notch; the jig is removed and the cut is

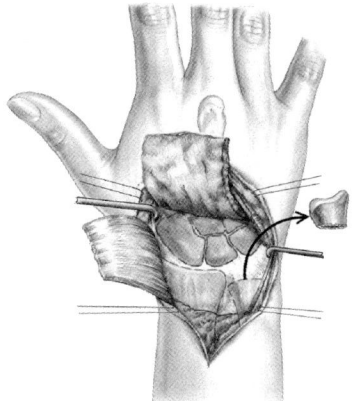

Fig. 2. Exposure of the distal radius and carpus using a radially based retinacular flap and distally based capsular flap. Ulnar head excision is optional.

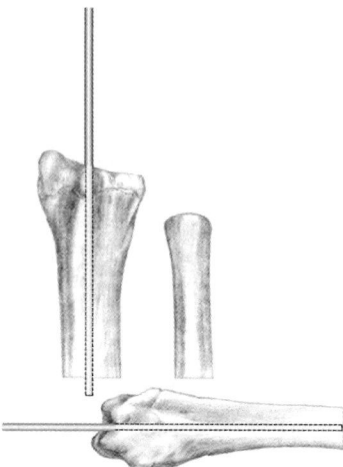

Fig. 3. A guide rod inserted to align cutting block and broach for radius preparation.

completed with the saw by free-hand technique wherby it flares slightly ulnarward and out through the distal articular surface of the radius. The cutting block and pins are removed, the guide rod reinserted, and the appropriate sized intramedullary broach is mounted on the rod. The broach is aligned with the sigmoid notch and dorsal rim of the radius and driven into the radius until its collar becomes flush with the cortex. (Fig. 5) A trial radial component is inserted. The carpus can be reduced on the radial component to assess soft tissue tension. If it is excessive, further resection of the radius may be necessary but is usually delayed until the carpal preparation is completed. In preparing the carpus, the scaphoid and triquetrum are temporarily pinned if they are mobile to facilitate the osteotomy. The lunate is excised by sharp dissection or rongeur. Using the drill guide, a hole is made in the center of the capitate. The carpal guide bar is inserted in the hole. The carpal cutting block is applied and positioned to resect the proximal 1mm of hamate, a

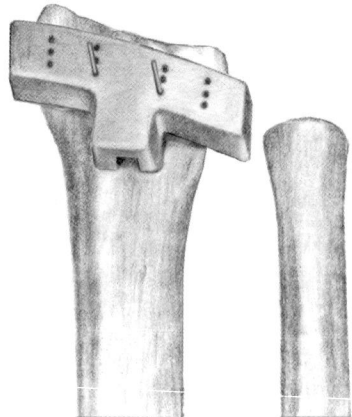

Fig. 4. Radial cutting block is applied to resect the articular surface at the proper angle.

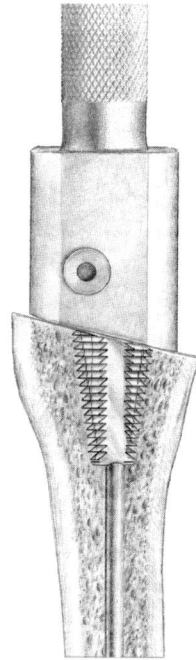

Fig. 5. Radius is broached using a cannulated broach over a guide rod.

small amount of the capitate head, and about half of the scaphoid and triquetrum. (Fig. 6) The cutting block is held with temporary fixation pins. The osteotomy is made with a small oscillating saw.

The trial carpal component is inserted and the holes for the screws are made using the drill guide. The radial drill hole passes through the scaphoid, trapezium, and second CMC joint to a depth of 30–35 mm (Fig. 7). The hole is typically not perpendicular to the carpal component, but the screws and the component are designed to accommodate oblique

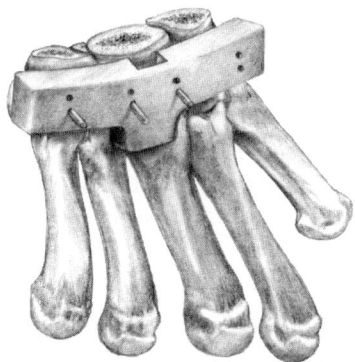

Fig. 6. A carpal cutting block is applied to guide the osteotomy through the capitate head, scaphoid waist, and midtriquetrum.

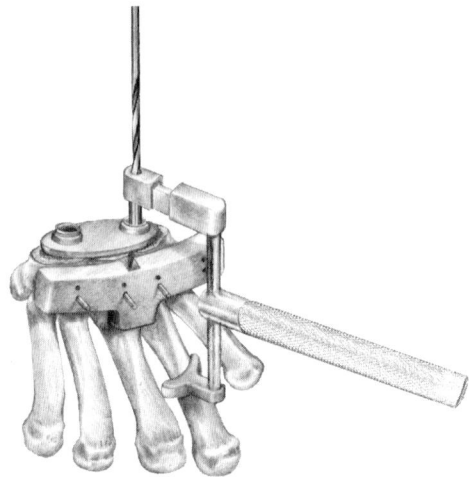

Fig. 7. Trial carpal component is inserted and holes are made for the screws using a special drill guide.

screw angles. Again using the drill guide, the ulnar hole is made into the hamate to a depth of 15–20 mm, but does not cross the mobile CMC joint.

The trial screws for the carpal component are inserted and the trial poly component is applied. The prosthesis is reduced and its motion and stability are tested. It is typically quite stable and should demonstrate approximately 35° of flexion and 35° of extension with modest tightness at full extension. If the volar capsule is limiting extension, the radius may need to be shortened slightly (2 mm). When a preoperative flexion contracture is present, a step-cut tendon lengthening of the wrist flexors may be necessary. Conversely, if tension is insufficient, the palmar joint capsule is inspected and repaired when detached. However, if the capsule is intact, a thicker polyethylene may be required.

Prior to implanting the final prosthesis, three horizontal mattress sutures of 2-0 polyester are placed through small bone holes along the dorsal rim of the distal radius for eventual capsule closure. If the ulnar head was resected, also place sutures through the dorsal neck. The articular surfaces are removed from the triquetrum, capitate, hamate, scaphoid, and trapezoid and previously resected bone is packed into the spaces to achieve an intercarpal arthrodesis. The final implants are impacted into place and the final screws are inserted tightly. The capsule should be repaired to completely enclose the implants. The extensor retinaculum is repaired leaving the extensor carpi radialis longus and brevis and the extensor pollicis longus superficial to the retinaculum. The skin is closed over a self-suction drain, and a volar plaster wrist splint is applied.

6. Postoperative management

The postoperative dressing and plaster splint are removed day 2 and a supervised exercise program is begun, including full digital motion and gentle active wrist motion (flexion, extension, radial and ulnar deviation, pronation, supination). Wrist extension is specifically emphasized. Strengthening is added at week 4 and full activities permitted after 8 weeks. The patient is advised to avoid impact loading of the wrist (e.g., use of a hammer, playing tennis) and repetitive forceful use of the hand. In general, patients are advised to only intermittently lift greater than 10 lb.

7. Results

In Menon's first report of 37 Universal prostheses with a mean follow-up of 6.7 years (range 4 to 10 years), no case demonstrated radiographic evidence of distal component loosening [18]. In a further follow-up study that included 57 implants, carpal component loosening was again not reported [23]. Subsidence of the radial component was observed but was not progressive or symptomatic. Similar to other prostheses, the Universal implant provided consistently good pain relief (90%) and a functional range of motion. Average postoperative motion was 36° extension, 41° flexion, 7° radial deviation, and 13° ulnar deviation. Dislocation was the most common complication, with 5 occurring in the first 37 cases and a total of 6 among the 57 cases in the later follow-up.

A prospective study of 22 Universal prosthesis implanted by two surgeons with a 1 to 2 year follow up demonstrated results similar to Menon's. Patients achieved an average of 41° flexion and 35° extension [20]. Disabilities of the Arm, Shoulder, and Hand (DASH) outcome survey scores improved 24 points at 2 years. Three prostheses (14%) were unstable and required further treatment; all three were in patients with highly active rheumatoid disease with severe wrist laxity. A further multicenter study of 53 patients again showed good results at 1 to 5 year follow up with nearly equivalent outcomes of motion and patient satisfaction achieved by all surgeons [24]. Dislocation continued to occur with a 9% overall incidence. Distal component loosening has occurred in four patients, all of whom had persistently active synovitis and failed to achieve an intercarpal fusion resulting in lack of solid bony implant support.

Early results with the Universal 2 prosthesis in 25 patients (20 women and 5 men) operated by two surgeons have been excellent. Twenty patients had rheumatoid arthritis, 2 post-traumatic arthritis, and 3 osteoarthritis. All prostheses were implanted uncemented. Results revealed excellent fixation with an average of 37° flexion, 33° extension, 22° ulnar deviation and 9° radial deviation. Pain relief was rated good by all patients but mild ulnar sided wrist discomfort persisted in 5. Pain relief and motion often did not reach their maximum improvements for 6 months. Average DASH scores improved 20% and PRWE scores improved 35%. No cases showed radiographic implant loosening, but one osteopenic patient had 3 mm of subsidence which plateaued. There have been no dislocations and no implant loosenings or revisions [25]. An additional surgeon survey found no reported dislocations or revisions in over 125 wrists implanted in the United States.

In the initial group of 20 patients, the carpal component stem fractured in three patients between the first and second year post-operatively who had the first version of this implant. The carpal component was subsequently redesigned with a greater diameter and stronger stem as well as full porous coating over its entire distal surface (stem and plate) for better durability and osteointegration. No fractures have been found with the revised version of the carpal component.

8. Potential complications

Potential intra-operative complications include fractures and tendon injury, both of which can be treated at that time. Possible postoperative complications include wound healing problems (hematoma, wound edge necrosis, dehiscence), extensor tendon adhesions, wrist stiffness, wrist imbalance, distal radioulnar joint problems (impingement, instability, arthrosis), prosthetic instability, aseptic loosening, and infection. The true incidence of these complications is unknown for the newest designs of wrist replacement currently in use, but appears to be low during the first 2 years post-operative. With the exceptions of advanced loosening and infection, each of these complications is treated based on the perspective of the patients needs and desires.

9. Failed TWA

Revision arthroplasty, arthrodesis and resection arthroplasty are options for salvaging a failed total wrist arthroplasty due to imbalance, loosening or instability [26]. Revision arthroplasty is an option for aseptic loosening if there is adequate bone stock or if bone grafting is feasible. The thickened capsule must be widely released to allow wrist flexion and extraction of the components. If there has been substantial subsidence, lengthening of the wrist flexors and extensor tendons may be required. Iliac crest bone graft may be needed to fill defects and re-establish the basic architecture of the carpus. When using the Universal 2 prosthesis for revision, the graft can be transfixed to the remaining carpus using the carpal component fixation screws. Since the decision to perform a revision depends primarily on the integrity of the bone and soft-tissues, it may not be possible to decide until direct inspection at the time of surgery. Thus, the surgeon must be prepared for both arthroplasty and arthrodesis. Patients with poor bone stock, severe capsule defects, or particulate synovitis are rarely indicated for revision arthroplasty. An established infection should be treated by implant removal and either primary or delayed conversion to an arthrodesis [8,27].

10. Conclusion

Total wrist arthroplasty preserves motion and improves hand function for daily tasks and lower demand vocational and avocational activities. It is often preferable to fusion when both wrists are arthritic. Newer prosthetic designs provide a functional range of motion, better wrist balance, reduced risk of loosening, and better implant stability than older designs. The success of total wrist arthroplasty depends on appropriate patient selection, careful preoperative planning, and sound surgical technique.

References

[1] M.J. Goodman, et al., Arthroplasty of the rheumatoid wrist with silicone rubber: an early evaluation, J. Hand Surg. [Am.] 5 (2) (1980) 114–121.
[2] A.J. Vicar, R.I. Burton, Surgical management of the rheumatoid wrist-fusion or arthroplasty, J. Hand Surg. [Am.] 11 (6) (1986) 790–797.

[3] A.B. Swanson, Flexible implant arthroplasty for arthritic disabilities of the radiocarpal joint. A silicone rubber intramedullary stemmed flexible hinge implant for the wrist joint, Orthop. Clin. North Am. 4 (2) (1973) 383–394.

[4] S.L. Jolly, et al., Swanson silicone arthroplasty of the wrist in rheumatoid arthritis: a long-term follow-up, J. Hand Surg. [Am.] 17 (1) (1992) 142–149.

[5] J.F. Fatti, A.K. Palmer, J.F. Mosher, The long-term results of Swanson silicone rubber interpositional wrist arthroplasty, J. Hand Surg. [Am.] 11 (2) (1986) 166–175.

[6] J.K. Stanley, A.R. Tolat, Long-term results of Swanson silastic arthroplasty in the rheumatoid wrist, J. Hand Surg. [Br.] 18 (3) (1993) 381–388.

[7] C.A. Peimer, et al., Reactive synovitis after silicone arthroplasty, J. Hand Surg. [Am.] 11 (5) (1986) 624–638.

[8] D.C. Ferlic, S.N. Jolly, M.L. Clayton, Salvage for failed implant arthroplasty of the wrist, J. Hand Surg. [Am.] 17 (5) (1992) 917–923.

[9] H. Meuli, Total wrist arthroplasty. Experience with a noncemented wrist prosthesis, Clin. Orthop. 342 (1997) 77–83.

[10] D.A. Dennis, D.C. Ferlic, M.L. Clayton, Volz total wrist arthroplasty in rheumatoid arthritis: a long-term review, J. Hand Surg. [Am.] 11 (4) (1986) 483–490.

[11] J. Menon, Total wrist replacement using the modified Volz prosthesis, J. Bone Joint Surg., Am. 69 (7) (1987) 998–1006.

[12] M.P. Figgie, et al., Trispherical total wrist arthroplasty in rheumatoid arthritis, J. Hand Surg. [Am.] 15 (2) (1990) 217–223.

[13] T.K. Cobb, R.D. Beckenbaugh, Biaxial total-wrist arthroplasty, J. Hand Surg. [Am.] 21 (6) (1996) 1011–1021.

[14] T.K. Cobb, R.D. Beckenbaugh, Biaxial long-stemmed multipronged distal components for revision/bone deficit total-wrist arthroplasty, J. Hand Surg. [Am.] 21 (5) (1996) 764–770.

[15] S. Radmer, R. Andresen, M. Sparmann, Wrist arthroplasty with a new generation of prostheses in patients with rheumatoid arthritis, J. Hand Surg. [Am.] 24 (5) (1999) 935–943.

[16] M. Rizzo, R.D. Beckenbaugh, Results of biaxial total wrist arthroplasty with a modified (long) metacarpal stem, J. Hand Surg. [Am.] 28 (4) (2003) 577–584.

[17] S. Radmer, R. Andresen, M. Sparmann, Total arthroplasty in patients with rheumatoid arthritis, J. Hand Surg. [Am.] 28 (5) (2003) 789–794.

[18] J. Menon, Universal Total Wrist Implant: experience with a carpal component fixed with three screws, J. Arthroplast. 13 (5) (1998) 515–523.

[19] N.M. Grosland, R.D. Rogge, B.D. Adams, Influence of Articular Geometry on Prosthetic Wrist Stability, Clin. Orthop. 412 (2004) 134–142.

[20] B.J. Divelbiss, C. Sollerman, B.D. Adams, Early results of the Universal total wrist arthroplasty in rheumatoid arthritis, J. Hand Surg. [Am.] 27 (2) (2002) 195–204.

[21] H. Hastings, Total wrist arthrodesis for post traumatic conditions, Ind. Hand Cent. Newsl. 1 (1994) 14–18.

[22] L.H. Millender, E.A. Nalebuff, Arthrodesis of the rheumatoid wrist. An evaluation of sixty patients and a description of a different surgical technique, J. Bone Joint Surg., Am. 55 (5) (1973) 1026–1034.

[23] J. Menon, Total wrist arthroplasty for rheumatoid arthritis, in: A.P. Safer P, G. Goucher (Eds.), Current Practice in Hand Surgery, Martin Dunitz, London, England, 1997, pp. 209–214.

[24] B.D. Adams, A multicenter study of the universal total wrist prosthesis, 57th Annual Meeting of the American Society for Surgery of the Hand, Phoenix, Arizona, 2002.

[25] B.D. Adams, Universal 2 total wrist arthroplasty, 55th Annual Meeting of the Association of Bone and Joint Surgeons, 2003, [Paris, France].

[26] M.P. Lorei, et al., Failed total wrist arthroplasty. Analysis of failures and results of operative management, Clin. Orthop. (342) (1997) 84–93.

[27] W.P. Cooney III, R.D. Beckenbaugh, R.L. Linscheid, Total wrist arthroplasty. Problems with implant failures, Clin. Orthop. (187) (1984) 121–128.

International Congress Series 1295 (2006) 94–106

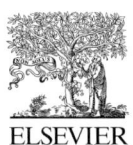

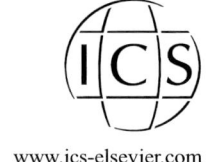

www.ics-elsevier.com

Options in extensor tendon reconstruction in rheumatoid arthritis

S. Schindele [a,b,*], D. Kloss [b], D. Herren [a]

[a] Hand Center, Schulthess Clinic, Zurich, Switzerland
[b] Department Hand-, Plastic and Reconstructive Surgery Kantonsspital St.Gallen, Switzerland

Abstract. There is a decreased incidence of extensor tendon rupture in rheumatoid arthritis due to progress in drug therapy with the consequence that destructive tenosynovitis occurs less often. However, in the long-term course of the disease, the tendons will tend to show signs of attrition at the sharp bone margins as, for example, in caput ulnae syndrome or at Lister's tubercle. Tendon rupture usually begins ulnarly, progressing over the wrist and extending radially, therefore, the causes of attrition must be remedied to prevent further ruptures. Generally, tendon reconstruction will no longer be possible by primary end-to-end suture at this stage. As the number of ruptures increases, various techniques such as side-to-side suture fixation, tendon transfers or tendon grafting are employed. These techniques will be described below. © 2006 Elsevier B.V. All rights reserved.

Keywords: Rheumatoid arthritis; Extensor tendon rupture; Extensor tendon reconstruction; Tendon graft; Tendon transfer

1. Introduction

Rheumatoid arthritis is essentially a disease of the synovial membrane with all its consequences. The tendon sheaths lined with synovial tissue that surround the tendons in the region of the hand and wrist may be involved in the rheumatoid process as well as the synovial membranes of the joints. Tenosynovitis in the context of rheumatoid arthritis occurs frequently and may become manifest months before signs of joint involvement are identified [1–3].

Although there has been an awareness of spontaneous tendon rupture for a long time, it was Vaughan-Jackson who in 1948 [4] drew attention to the importance of tendinous

* Corresponding author. Schulthess Clinic, Handcenter, Lengghalde 2, CH-8008 Zurich, Switzerland. Tel.: +41 44 385 7488; fax: +41 44 385 7232.
E-mail address: stephan.schindele@kws.ch (S. Schindele).

0531-5131/ © 2006 Elsevier B.V. All rights reserved.
doi:10.1016/j.ics.2006.03.030

alterations with reference to two cases of spontaneous rupture of the extensor tendons at the level of the distal radioulnar joint (DRUJ). This was followed by an increasing number of reports on the pathology of the tendons in rheumatoid arthritis. Investigations undertaken by Kellgern and Ball [5] revealed that the tendons were affected by typical changes in over 50% of cases.

Synovitic involvement of the extensor tendons have been observed more frequently than for the flexor tendons in the hand. Mannsat [6] diagnosed dorsal tenosynovitis in 30% of his patients as opposed to only 22% on the palmar surface. It is also of note that the abductor pollicis longus (APL) and extensor pollicis brevis (EPB) tendons were rarely affected in the region of the first extensor compartment.

The clinical picture of rheumatoid tenosynovitis depends on its localization. In the majority of cases, tenosynovitis causes pain whereby spontaneous tendon rupture can be an entirely painless event. Primarily, synovitis tends only to affect the mobile tissue of the tendon sheath. During the course of the disease the tendon is infiltrated and ultrastructural changes take place in the tendinous tissue, which may include ischemic necroses, this may lead to loss of function and eventually rupture even without additional mechanical irritation [7]. Progress has clearly been made in the treatment of rheumatoid arthritis in recent years due to the further development and improvement of remedial medication. Drug therapy has had a particularly positive effect on the treatment of tenosynovitis such that this condition has taken a back seat and spontaneous tendon rupture has become less common.

Today the main cause of spontaneous rupture of the extensor tendons at the wrist is attrition of the tendons over an eroded bony prominence. This type of attrition is seen predominantly in the region of the ulnar head and Lister's tubercle. The tubercle forms a bony deflection sheave for the extensor pollicis longus tendon, which is subject to increased mechanical load accordingly.

The head of the ulna, adjacent to which lie the ulnar extensor digitorum tendons, dislocates dorsally if there is instability of the DRUJ and supination deformity of the carpus, and likewise forms a deflection sheave for the adjacent tendons. Surgical intervention aims to eliminate this potential cause of rupture. As a rule, rupture has been

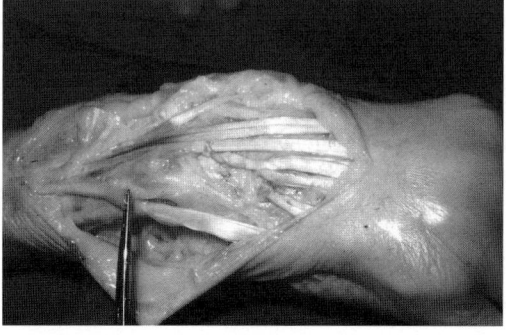

Fig. 1. Right hand: Caput ulnae-syndrome with dorsal dislocation of the eroded ulna head causes attrition and rupture of EDQ and EDC[4+5].

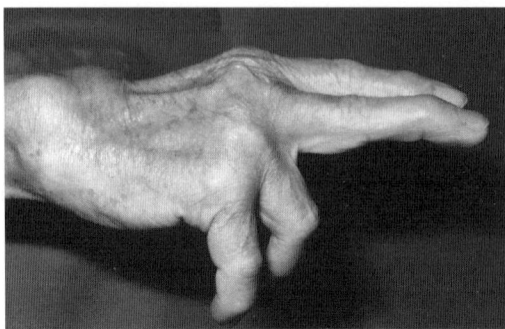

Fig. 2. Right hand: Clinical presentation of EDQ and EDC[4+5] rupture with synovitis and dorsal dislocation of the ulna head (caput ulnae-syndrome). Intraoperativ see Fig. 1.

caused by attrition of the tendon over the dorsally protruding ulnar head (caput ulnae syndrome) (see Fig. 1). In most cases, resection of the head of the distal ulna alone is sufficient (Darrach procedure). If radiology suggests possible radiocarpal instability according to Simmens classification, arthrodesis of the DRUJ (Sauve–Kapandji procedure) should be preferred with a view to radiocarpal partial arthrodesis, [8,9].

2. Diagnosis

Spontaneous extensor tendon ruptures are usually painless and become manifest after minor injury or during normal use of the hand. The prerequisites for prompt, correct diagnosis are therefore an attentive patient and a treating physician with the relevant knowledge. The initial presentation is sudden loss of ability to extend one or more fingers (see Fig. 2). Patients with rheumatoid arthritis are accustomed to functional limitations and disabilities associated with their illness. Therefore, they tend to play down this insidious functional deterioration. They only seek medical advice if the loss of function becomes very apparent and the restrictions become subjectively relevant. Isolated ruptures of the extensor digiti quinti (EDQ) and the extensor pollicis longus (EPL) only cause very slight functional loss which is often overlooked by the patient or masked by other more severe deformities.

The etiological factors that lead to rupture of individual tendons will often be followed by other tendon ruptures if left uncorrected. All too often rupture of the EDQ goes unnoticed and is followed by rupture of the extensor digitorum communis (EDC) of the ring and middle fingers. As a rule the long finger extensors rupture from ulnar to radial leaving the tendons of the extensor indices intact. Most frequently rupture is caused when the tendon has become frayed due to mechanical abrasion over a sharp bony prominence in the region of the ulnar wrist joint and/or the head of the ulna (see above).

3. Differential diagnosis

Although the sudden inability to extend the small, ring and middle fingers is generally the result of rupture of the relevant tendons, the differential diagnosis should exclude three other possible conditions that may also present as extensor insufficiency of these fingers:

1. Palmar dislocation or subluxation of the metacarpophalangeal joint (MCP) is characterized by both active and passive loss of joint extension. The active tension in the extensors is however usually palpable.
2. Active loss of joint extension in the MCP joints may also occur when the extensors have dislocated in an ulnar direction into the space between the heads of the metacarpals. If the extensor tendon is displaced too far on the palmar side of the central axis of the MCP joint, it will act as a flexor. The condition is easily diagnosed if the patient can actively stabilize the passively extended MCP joints.
3. Compression of the posterior interosseous and/or radial nerve [10]: Patients with radial paresis in the region of the proximal radioulnar joint demonstrate a tendency towards radial deviation of the wrist due to paralysis of the extensor carpi ulnaris (ECU). Synovitis of the elbow joint with involvement of the proximal radioulnar joint may indicate a neurogenic etiology. The most reliable sign is however a positive tenodesis effect in the region of the MCP joints. If secondary extension of the MCP joints occurs during passive wrist flexion, then the continuity of the common extensor tendons is proven. EMG diagnosis may be relevant in cases of arthrodesis or ankylosis of the wrist.

4. Technique of extensor tendon reconstruction

4.1. Rupture of extensor pollicis longus (EPL)

Rupture of the EPL tendon in the context of rheumatoid arthritis is a frequent event. However, the functional loss caused by it can differ greatly and depend essentially on the functionality of the intact extensor pollicis brevis (EPB) and the status of the joints of the first ray. EPL rupture is often characterized by active functional loss at the interphalangeal joint (IP) but more frequently there is a reduction of extension strength and extension of the MCP joint as the EPB is too weak to preserve the full extension capability of the MCP joint. Furthermore, the intrinsic muscles will also contribute to extension of the IP joint. This is one reason why EPL rupture is frequently overlooked.

Restoration of EPL function is recommended if there is severe functional disability. In principle, reconstruction is possible by means of end-to-end suture, graft or tendon transfer. End-to-end suture is generally no longer possible, even immediately after rupture. This applies to all spontaneous rheumatic tendon ruptures. Tendon grafts that have been woven through tissue altered by inflammatory processes tend to adhere and, therefore, are not necessarily recommended for the repair of spontaneously ruptured extensor tendons in the rheumatoid hand. Nevertheless, given that a contractile muscle is still intact, reconstruction of the EPL by graft technique can lead to a good clinical outcome because the powerful flexor pollicis longus (FPL) will, in the long-term, counteract tendon adhesions.

Transfer operations are generally preferred for the restoration of EPL function. The most frequently used structures are the tendon of the extensor indicis proprius (EIP) or, less often, the tendons of the ECRL or EDQ. Nalebuff [11] prefers EIP transfer for the following reasons: The EIP tendon can be released at the MCP joint without any apparent functional loss for this joint. Rather surprisingly, the patient does not lose the ability to extend the index finger independently from the other long fingers. Strength and amplitude of the EIP are almost identical to those of the EPL [12,13]. If there is rupture of at least two ulnar extensor tendons in addition to EPL rupture, then the EIP is less available because it is required for ulnar reconstruction. In these cases, the reconstruction technique of choice will be a palmaris longus graft. If the palmaris longus is missing, a strip of ECRL, plantaris or extensor tendon of the 4th toe may serve as transplant material. However, tendon grafting is only appropriate for recent ruptures where there is good contractility of the proximal tendon muscle unit.

If the rupture has existed for a longer period, transfer of EPL to the EPB will be appropriate [14]. In this procedure, the distal stump of the EPL is transferred end-to-side to the EPB over the first metacarpal (see Fig. 3). Clinically, only simultaneous extension of the interphalangeal and MCP joints is retained, which amounts to only a slight functional restriction.

Nalebuff warns against transfer of the radial wrist extensors (ECRL or ECRB) which might affect the tendon balance of the wrist. Since it is not unusual for the ulnar finger extensors to be affected by rupture as well, it is better to refrain from transferring the EDQ from ulnar to radial.

4.2. Rupture of one long finger extensor tendon

Rupture of a single long finger extensor can affect any finger, but the small finger is frequently affected the most. The extent of active extension loss at the MCP joint of the small finger depends on whether only the EDQ or both the EDQ and the EDC-5 are ruptured. Isolated rupture of the EDQ tends to cause only slight loss of active extension at the MCP joint and almost always remains unnoticed. The relevant function test requires that the patient stretch the small finger with the fist clenched. This blocks the action of the EDC-5. An extension deficit of 30–40° will be observed if the EDQ is dysfunctional.

Reconstruction of the EDQ tendon is most easily achieved by end-to-side suture of the distal tendon stump to the adjacent tendons of EDC-5 or EDC-4 (see Fig. 4). Correct initial tension is essential for a good result. The tenodesis effect seen intraoperatively during movement of the wrist must allow all four fingers to be moved simultaneously.

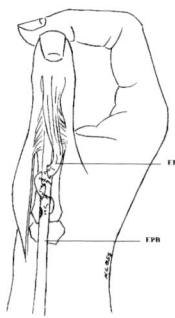

Fig. 3. Restoration of IP extension in the thumb can be achieved by transferring the EPL to the EPB over the first metacarpal.

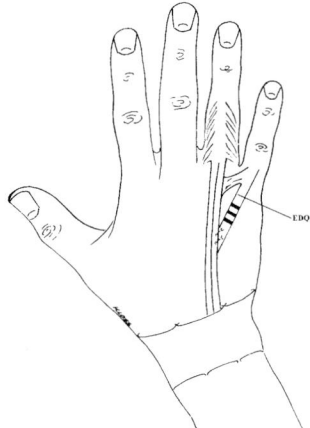

Fig. 4. Restoration of little finger extension by end-to-side suture technique of the EDQ to the adjacent tendons of EDC$^{4/5}$.

Another possibility for primary tendon transfer is to place the EIP tendon into the tendon stump of the small finger extensors (EDQ/EDC-5). Before commencing this procedure, the integrity of EDC-2 must be assessed so that the extension of the index finger is not jeopardized. The EIP tendon is located on the ulnar side of the EDC-2 tendon and both pass through the 4th extensor compartment with the EDC tendons. Since the muscle belly is situated very distally, it can easily be differentiated from the EDC tendons. Transfer is achieved by weaving in the tendon stump in a Pulvertaft technique (see Fig. 5). It is important to maintain adequate tension to facilitate postoperative stretching. Intraoperatively, the small finger should achieve somewhat greater extension at the MCP joint than the ring finger. Complete passive fist closure should be possible with the wrist in 30–40° extension.

4.3. Rupture of two long finger extensors (EDQ/EDC-5 + EDC-4)

Side-to-side suture of both distal tendon stumps to the EDC3 tendon is an inadequate solution to the problem. On the one hand, the strength of the middle finger is hardly sufficient to achieve full extension of the 3 ulnar fingers and, on the other, the stump of the small finger tendon is often so short that any suture technique is hampered.

In this case, side-to-side suture of the distal tendon stump of the ruptured EDC4 tendon to the intact tendon of the middle finger only is recommended. Tendon grafting or EIP transfer can be performed to restore extension to the small finger (see Fig. 6). In addition

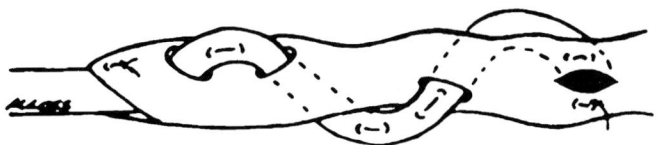

Fig. 5. Pulvertaft-technique. Secure tendon connection can be achieved by weaving in the tendon stumps 3 to 4 times in a 90° angled technique.

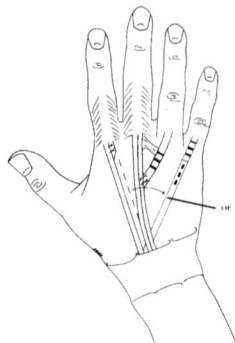

Fig. 6. Restoration of little and ring finger extension by end-to-side suture technique of the EDC⁴ to EDC³ and EIP transfer to EDQ.

to reports of EIP tendon transfer, transfer of the wrist extensors has also been described. However, transfer of the extensor carpi ulnaris (ECU) is a less appropriate procedure since this tendon is important to wrist stability and its removal could produce radial rotation of the wrist. Furthermore, the wrist extensors have less excursion than the finger extensors so that limited flexion or insufficient extension after transfer can occur.

Although reconstruction with a free tendon transplant may be problematic due to the risk of secondary adhesions [15], good outcomes have been described for this technique [16–18]. The precondition is that the contractility of the relevant muscles is still intact, therefore, there is a time limit on this technique. Possible donors for tendon graft are the palmaris longus, strips of ECRL or ECRB, also plantaris and the extensor tendon of the fourth toe. Intraoperatively, the grafts should be maintained under relatively high tension and stabilized by weave sutures in order to compensate for the anticipated elongation of the muscles. If muscle fibrosis with limited contractility is already present and tension is too high but the extensibility of the fingers is good, functional deficit may result due to loss of finger flexion. Nakamura [19] therefore recommends that tendon grafting should not be performed if there is a contractile proximal muscle–tendon unit and reduced passive excursion of less than 2 cm becomes apparent intraoperatively.

4.4. Rupture of three long finger extensors (EDQ/EDC-5 + EDC-4 + EDC-3)

In the case of rupture of the extensors of the small, ring and middle fingers, tendon grafting can be performed as a means of reconstruction as for the rupture of only two extensors. As already mentioned above, this should only be considered for recent loss of extensor function.

Extension losses that have existed for a long time should be treated by tendon transfer because of the lack of contractility of the proximal tendon–muscle unit.

If the EDC-2 tendon is intact then the distal EDC-3 tendon stump can be sutured end-to-side to it. Restoration of function to the small and ring fingers is achieved by EIP transfer to the tendon stumps of EDC-4, EDC-5 and EDQ (see Fig. 7). If the EDC-2 of the index finger is also ruptured and only the EIP is intact, then the latter is not available as a tendon graft donor. In this case, transfer of the flexor digitorum superficialis of the ring

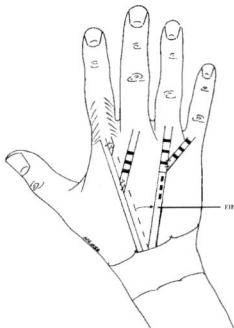

Fig. 7. Restoration of little, ring and middle finger extension by end-to-side suture technique of the EDC^3 to EDC^2 and EIP transfer to $EDQ/EDC^{4/5}$.

finger to the distal tendon stumps of EDC-4/5 and EDQ should be carried out and extension of the middle finger restored by side-to-side suture to the EIP tendon.

4.5. Rupture of all finger extensors (EDQ/EDC-5 + EDC-4 + EDC-3 + EDC-2/EIP)

As for the procedures described above, a bridge graft may be useful to repair rupture of all four long finger extensors. Here the same conditions apply as given above with regard to time of operation and donor tendons. An additional consideration is that as the number of grafts increases so does the probability of insufficiency, therefore, the decision to reconstruct with tendon graft alone should be taken with caution.

If rupture of four or more extensors has occurred, transfer of the EIP in combination with side-to-side sutures will no longer be sufficient; the strength of the reconstruction would not be enough to activate all four long finger extensors. The only possible donor tendons are the flexor digitorum superficialis tendons (FDS) of the ring and middle fingers. This technique was originally described by Boyes [20] for the treatment of radial nerve palsy. The superficialis tendon is detached from the distal palm and passed through the interosseous membrane from the flexor to the extensor side. It is important that the tendon should pass as directly as possible through an adequately large aperture in the interosseous membrane. Nalebuff and Patel [21] modified the technique so that the superficialis tendon is not threaded through the interosseous membrane but is passed radially around the radius in a dorsal direction (see Fig. 8). Ulnar deflection is also possible, although not recommended as it may promote ulnar shift of the wrist and fingers. Scarring proximal to the wrist and in the region of the interosseous membrane makes a radial deflection of the tendon seem preferable, whereby radial pull on the tendons also tends to favour ulnar drift of the fingers and the wrist. Up to three extensor tendons can be powered by one superficialis tendon. However, if there is rupture of all the long finger tendons then transfer of two superficialis tendons is required. Extension of the ring and middle fingers can be restored with the FDS-4 tendon, and extension of the index and middle fingers can be reconstructed with the FDS-3 tendon. It is important that the integrity of the relevant deep flexor tendons (FDP-3, FDP-4) is assessed prior to detachment to ensure that excision will not lead to a flexion deficit.

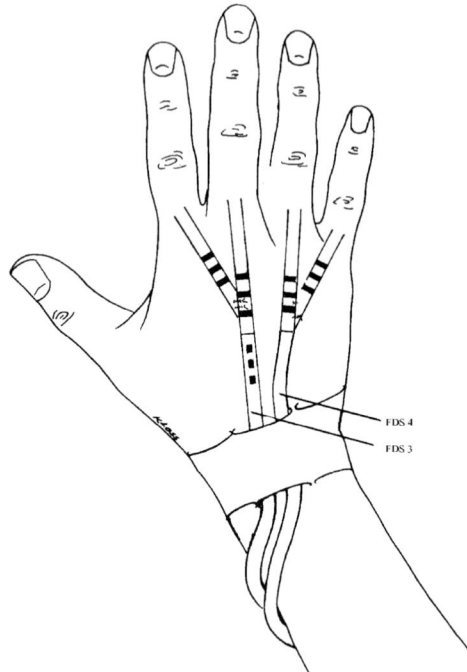

Fig. 8. Restoration of all long finger extensors by radially passed tendon transfer of the FDS[3] to index and middle finger and FDS[4] to ring and little finger extensor stumps.

The operation is performed through three skin incisions. The first straight incision is made dorsally over the wrist, the extensor tendon ruptures are visualized and tendons trimmed back until normal tendon tissue is identified. The protruding dorsal bone margins have to be smoothed and usually the ulnar head has to be resected. Any work on the bone should be completed before tendon transfer to eliminate the risk of renewed tendon attrition. A longitudinal incision is made on the palmar aspect of the wrist proximal to the flexion crease and the relevant muscle–tendon units of the FDS-3 and FDS-4 are identified. Then a transverse incision is made in the flexion crease of the MCP joints and the relevant superficialis tendon is divided and brought forward to the more proximal incision. The tendons are then taken subcutaneously on the radial side in a dorsal direction under the branches of the radial nerve and woven into the appropriate extensor tendon by means of weave suture. It is crucial for the functional outcome that the correct level of tension is achieved. This must be strong enough to compensate for future elongation stresses. If tension is adequate, a tenodesis effect will result when the wrist is moved.

4.6. Rupture of the wrist extensors (ECRL, ECRB, ECU)

Rupture of the wrist extensors on the radial (ECRL/ECRB) and ulnar (ECU) aspects is rarely seen. There are no reports in the literature of isolated ruptures in an otherwise radiologically normal wrist. In most cases, radiological investigation reveals

Table 1
Recommended procedures in extensor tendon reconstruction in rheumatoid arthritis

Rupture	Side to side	Transfer	Graft
EPL	–	EIP or EPB (if EIP is needed for ulnar fingers)	Palmaris longus, ECRL/ECRB (only a strip) Extensor tendon 4.toe
EDQ	EDQ to EDC$^{4/5}$	EIP to EDQ	Palmaris longus, ECRL/ECRB (only a strip) Extensor tendon 4.toe
EDQ+EDC^5	EDQ/EDC^5 to EDC^4	EIP to EDQ/EDC^5	Palmaris longus, ECRL/ECRB (only a strip) Extensor tendon 4.toe
EDQ+EDC^{4+5}	EDC^4 to EDC^3 (and transfer)	EIP to EDQ/EDC^5	Palmaris longus, ECRL/ECRB (only a strip) Extensor tendon 4.toe
EDQ+EDC^{3+4+5}	EDC^3 to EDC^2 (and transfer)	EIP to EDQ/EDC^4	Palmaris longus, ECRL/ECRB (only a strip) Extensor tendon 4.toe
EDQ+EDC$^{2+3+4+5}$	EDC^3 to EIP (and transfer)	FDS^4 to EDQ/EDC^4	Palmaris longus, ECRL/ECRB (only a strip) Extensor tendon 4.toe
All 4 finger	–	FDS^4 to EDQ/EDC^4 and FDS^3 to EDC^{2+3}/EIP	Palmaris longus ECRL/ECRB (only a strip) Extensor tendon 4.toe
Thumb and all fingers	–	FDS^3 to EPL/EIP and FDS^4 to EDC$^{3-5}$	–

advanced arthritic destruction of the wrist and the MCP joints with concomitant rupture of several long finger extensors. In these cases, tendon transfer, e.g. brachioradialis, is of little value to restore mobility to the wrist, therefore, we would tend to recommend arthrodesis of the wrist with simultaneous reconstruction of the finger extensors only.

An overview of the most recommended procedures will be given in Table 1.

5. Postoperative care after extensor tendon reconstruction

It has proven valuable after surgical repair, whether it be tendon transfer, side-to-side repair or graft reconstruction, to apply a simple palmar postural splint with the wrist in extension (30–40°) and the MCP joints in slight flexion (10–20°) for the first few days postoperatively. This may be followed by further static treatment with the wrist and MCP joints in the positions just described for 3–4 more weeks. The PIP and DIP joints can be actively mobilized immediately. It is important that fist closure is confirmed within the first 3–4 weeks with the wrist in the fullest possible extension because an inability to achieve fist closure particularly of the ulnar rays indicates a functional restriction as opposed to a slight extension lag. Although dynamic splints to prevent adhesions may seem advantageous, they are not used very frequently. However, application of a dynamic splint may be beneficial in shielding double-sided weave sutures and preventing adhesions in those cases that have required several bridge grafts for the reconstruction of multiple extensor tendon ruptures.

6. Concomitant destruction of the wrist or MCP joints

Stiffness of the MCP joints will result if multiple extensor tendon ruptures combined with destruction of the MCP joints goes untreated for a long time. A necessary prerequisite

Table 2
Amplitude of different hand/forearm muscles for tendon transfer [22]

Muscle	Amplitude (cm)
Brachioradialis	3.0
FDP	7.0
FDS	6.5
EPL	6.0
EDC, EIP, EDQ	5.0
FPL	5.0
ECRL, ECRB, ECU, FCR,	3–4
Lumbicals	3.8
Interossei	2.0

for the restoration of extensor tendon function is an intact mobile MCP joint. Therefore, reconstruction of the MCP joints, that is to say, their passive mobility, should precede any tendon transfer surgery. A combination of MCP reconstruction by arthroplasty with simultaneous reconstruction of the extensors is possible. The most important issue here is not the method however, i.e. whether individual extensor tendon ruptures are treated by side-to-side suture, tendon graft or transfer, or whether superficialis transfer is performed for multiple ruptures.

Wrist arthroplasty can also be considered if there is severe concomitant destruction of the wrist but the wrist stabilizers are intact (ECRL, ECRB, ECU). The preservation of wrist mobility will have a positive influence on the finger extensors due to the tenodesis effect. Arthrodesis of the wrist should be performed if both sides are affected severely or in cases of reduced functional demands but also if simultaneous rupture of the wrist extensors has occurred. The subsequent reduction in mobility does lead to a reduction in the tenodesis effect but this is generally hardly noticeable in terms of function.

If the wrist is stiff due to arthrodesis or ankylosis, the wrist extensors (ECRL/ECRB) become available as donors for the reconstruction of multiple finger extensors. The disadvantage here is however not only the limited excursion of the wrist extensors but also their insufficient length. Direct suture repair with increased risk of rupture can be regarded as an alternative to an additional interpositional graft to lengthen the tendon. Whether it is

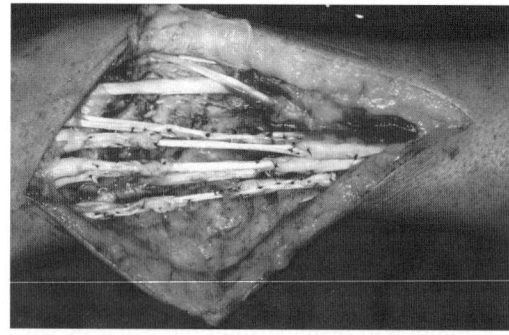

Fig. 9. Left hand: Tendon reconstruction of all four fingers by grafting.

better to take this risk or to perform EIP or superficialis transfer is a decision that has to be taken separately for each individual case.

7. Tendon transfer or tendon graft for the reconstruction of the finger extensors?

In theory, a good functional outcome will be achieved with either technique, therefore, the emphasis should be placed on the functional requirements of the patient, the concomitant disorders of the affected hand, and the personal experience of the surgeon.

The advantage of tendon transfer must be that only one suture site is required, thus there is a lesser risk of insufficient connectivity than would be the case for tendon graft which by definition has to bridge two suture sites. However, there is no data in the literature indicating which is best.

Another advantage of transfer is that it always provides a good and sufficient contractile muscle–tendon unit that permits powerful muscular traction, on the one hand, and sufficient amplitude for finger excursion to allow fist closure, on the other (see Table 2). Occasionally, however, functional restriction may result from detachment of the tendon and loss of the original function.

In contrast, reconstruction by tendon graft should only be performed if there is good contractility of the proximally migrated muscle–tendon unit. Since atrophy and muscle fibrosis sets in after retraction due to the temporary disuse of the muscle, the time to graft reconstruction should not exceed 12–20 weeks after rupture has occurred [18,19]. Nakamura and Katsuki [19] therefore recommends that contractility be assessed intraoperatively prior to reconstruction and that the idea of tendon grafting should be abandoned if there is a passive excursion of less than 2 cm. If a decision is taken to graft despite inadequate excursion and the patient's reduced functional requirements, the graft should not be woven into the ulnar finger rays under too much tension because this may lead to loss of fist closure. Generally the postoperative tip-to-palm distance correlates more closely with patient satisfaction then a restriction of extension. For this reason, tension in the reconstructed extensor tendon at the greatest possible dorsal extension of the wrist should permit passive finger flexion almost to fist closure since the possibility for postoperative stretching of the contracted muscle is very limited. However, in cases of good contractility good results can also be achieved with tendon grafting (see Figs. 9 and 10).

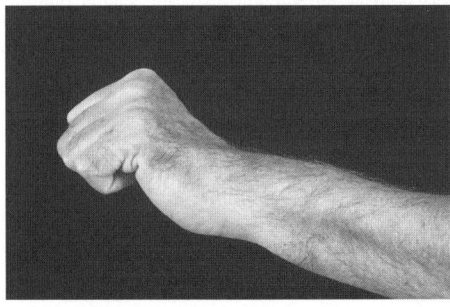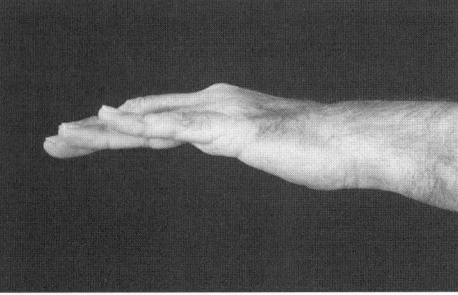

Fig. 10. Clinical result 6 months after the reconstruction with four intercalary grafts.

References

[1] J.H. Jakobs, E.V. Hess, I.P. Beswick, Rheumatoid arthritis presenting as tenosynovitis, J. Bone Jt. Surg., Br. 39 (1957) 288–292.

[2] A.G.L. Kay, Natural history of synovial hypertrophy in the rheumatoid hand, Ann. Rheum. Dis. 30 (1971) 98–102.

[3] E.A. Nalebuff, T.A. Potter, Rheumatoid involvement of tendon and tendon sheaths in the hand, Clin. Orthop. 59 (1968) 147–159.

[4] O.J. Vaughan-Jackson, Rupture of extensor tendons by attrition at the inferior radio-ulnar joint. Report of two cases, J. Bone Jt. Surg. 30-B (1948) 528–530.

[5] J.H. Kellgern, J. Ball, Tendon lesions in rheumatoid arthritis. A clinical–pathological study, Ann. Rheum. Dis. 9 (1950) 46–65.

[6] M. Mannsat, La main rheumatoide. Dissertation, Toulouse, 1970.

[7] M.F. Neurath, E. Stofft, Ultrastructure of the long flexor and extensor tendons of the hand in rheumatic tenosynovitis, Handchir. Mikrochir. Plast. Chir. 24 (1992) 159–164.

[8] B.R. Simmen, H. Huber, The wrist joint in chronic polyarthritis—a new classification based on the type of destruction in relation to the natural course and the consequences for surgical therapy, Handchir. Mikrochir. Plast. Chir. 26 (4) (1994) 182–189.

[9] M.P. Flury, D.B. Herren, B.R. Simmen, Rheumatoid arthritis of the wrist. Classification related to the natural course, Clin. Orthop. 366 (1999) 72–77.

[10] L. Marmor, J.F. Lawrence, E.L. Dubois, Posterior interosseous nerve palsy due to rheumatoid arthritis, J. Bone Jt. Surg., Am. 49 (1967) 381–383.

[11] E.A. Nalebuff, P.G. Feldo, L.H. Millender, Rheumatoid arthritis in the hand and wrist, in: D.P. Green (Ed.), Operative Hand Surgery, New York Churchill, Livingstone, 1988, pp. 1667–1677.

[12] E.Z. Browne, M.A. Teague, T.C. Snyder, Prevention of extensor lag after indicis proprius tendon transfer, J. Hand Surg. 4 (1979) 168–172.

[13] J.R. Moore, A.J. Weiland, L. Valdata, Independent index extension after extensor indicis proprius transfer, J. Hand Surg., Am. 12 (1987) 232–236.

[14] S. Harrison, A.J. Swannell, B.M. Ansel, Repair of extensor pollicis longus using extensor pollicis brevis in rheumatoid arthritis, Ann. Rheum. Dis. 31 (1972) 490–492.

[15] A.E. Flatt, in: A.E. Flatt (Ed.), The Care of Rheumatoid Hand, CV Mosby, St Louis, 1974, p. 114.

[16] F.W. Osterman Jr., et al., The treatment of ruptures of multiple extensor tendons at wrist level by a free tendon graft in the rheumatoid patient, J. Hand Surg. 12A (1987) 1038–1040.

[17] M. Minami, et al., Tendon ruptures in the rheumatoid hand, in: M. Vastamäki (Eds.), Current Trends in Hand Surgery, Elsevier Science B V, Amsterdam, 1995, pp. 515–521.

[18] J. Mountney, et al., Free tendon interposition grafting for the repair of ruptured extensor tendons in the rheumatoid hand, J. Hand Surg., Br. 23B (1998) 662–665.

[19] S. Nakamura, M. Katsuki, Tendon grafting for extensor tendon ruptures of fingers in rheumatoid hands, J. Hand Surg., Br. 27B (4) (2002) 326–328.

[20] J.H. Boyes, Bunnell's Surgery of the Hand, 5th edn., Lippincott, Philadelphia, 1970, p. 419.

[21] E.A. Nalebuff, M.R. Patel, Flexor digitorum sublimis transfer for multiple extensor tendon ruptures in rheumatoid arthritis, Plast. Reconstr. Surg. 52 (1973) 530–533.

[22] R.J. Smith, Principles of tendon transfers, in: R.J. Smith (Ed.), Tendon Transfers of the Hand and Forearm, Little, Brown and Co, Boston, 1987, pp. 13–34.

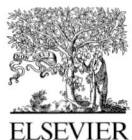

International Congress Series 1295 (2006) 107–117

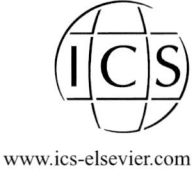

www.ics-elsevier.com

ELSEVIER

Flexor tendon synovectomy in rheumatoid arthritis

Philippe Saffar *

Institut Français de Chirurgie de la Main, 5, rue du Dôme, Paris 75116, France

Abstract. Rheumatoid hand deformities are often visible on the dorsal aspect of the hand and wrist. This explains why less attention has been given to the role of flexor tendon involvement in this condition. Swelling and joint distortions are also more visible on the dorsal aspect, although the sequences of movements, the major part of the joint and collateral ligaments, are volar. Hypertrophic synovitis is also more abundant and thicker volarly than dorsally. © 2006 Published by Elsevier B.V.

Keywords: Rheumatoid hand deformities; Flexor tendon involvement; Joint distortions; Hypertrophic synovitis

1. Introduction

In 1966, Smith et al. [1] have attracted attention to the deforming forces at the level of the MP joint and have concluded that the flexor tendons were a *predominant cause of deformities* (Figs. 1 and 2). Wise in 1975 [2] has confirmed that once the MP joint collateral ligaments are stretched by the ongoing rheumatoid process, flexor tendons exert a volar and ulnar force on the MP joint during grasping which causes the fingers to be pulled in a volar direction and creates fingers "ulnar drift".

Rheumatoid arthritis is basically a disease of the synovium and involves the synovial sheaths that surround the tendons at the level of hand and wrist. Proliferative synovitis infiltrates the tendons, causes formation of nodules, changes their ultrastructure, and eventually leads to spontaneous rupture.

* Tel.: +33 153655353; fax: +33 153655354.
  E-mail address: psaffar@ifcm.org.

0531-5131/ © 2006 Published by Elsevier B.V.
doi:10.1016/j.ics.2006.03.077

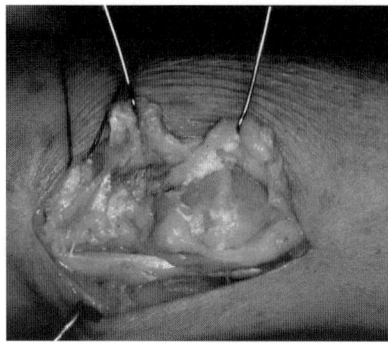

Fig. 1. Thick volar synovitis around flexor tendons.

The two principal symptoms of the disease on the volar aspect of the hand and wrist are

(1) Nerve compressions
    (a) Median nerve in the carpal tunnel: this may be the onset of the disease or an early symptom.
    (b) Ulnar nerve in Guyon's canal
(2) Flexor tenosynovitis

The diagnosis of flexor tenosynovitis remains a clinical diagnosis. Three main groups can be distinguished: isolated carpal tenosynovitis (20%), palmodigital tenosynovitis (50%), and diffuse tenosynovitis (30%). This synovitis may be seen on the volar aspect of

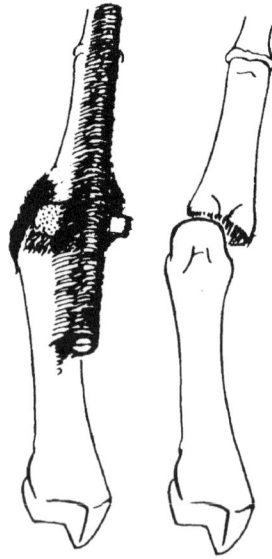

Fig. 2. Flexor tendons are a *predominant cause of the deformities*.

the hand: the palm and fingers are swollen. At the wrist, it may look like an hourglass with swelling proximal and distal to the carpal tunnel.

1.1. Clinical examination

Pain is always present, especially at night, and is a combination of inflammatory arthritis, synovitis and carpal tunnel syndrome symptoms.

1.1.1. At an early stage
Diagnosis is difficult:

- Flexor synovitis may be palpated or seen in the palm and wrist. It may also be present in the digital canal. Involvement of the fingers may be detected by crepitus when pressing volarly over the first phalanx during finger flexion. The second, third and fourth fingers are most frequently involved
  - trigger fingers and trigger wrist may be present;
  - finger motion is nearly normal and there is no obvious flexor tendon rupture;
  - there may be an onset of fingers ulnar drift, also caused by slackening of the flexor sheath. This can be detected on the radial side of the hand by pushing in an ulnar direction on the flexor tendons. This shift of the flexor tendons may also be palpated on the ulnar side of the second or third finger at its most proximal portion, the finger being flexed against resistance;
  - nerve compression may be among the first symptoms: numbness and tingling localized to the median nerve area, or less frequently than that of the ulnar nerve.

1.1.2. At an advanced stage

- a metacarpophalangeal (MP) volar subluxation may exist, mainly of the 2nd and 3rd fingers, with limitation of finger extension.
- the wrist may be radially deviated.
- flexor tenovitis is evident. Three different types of flexor tendon involvement are dis tinguished: isolated tenosynovitis, tenosynovitis with a tendon lesion and complete tendon rupture. During evolution, these different stages may coexist in the same patient. A clinical difference between tenosynovitis with and without a tendon lesion is not normally seen.

- Nodules are three times more frequent in the flexor tendons than the extensor tendons, and confined to the profundus tendon.
- Tendon rupture is evoked: the two causes of tendon ruptures are infiltration of the tendon by tenosynovitis and attrition by bony spurs. Ruptures are most often located at the wrist with the profundus tendon being most frequently affected. Cortisone injections may also have been an aggravating factor. Rupture may take place at the carpal tunnel or finger level.
- Finger motion is decreased (Fig. 3).

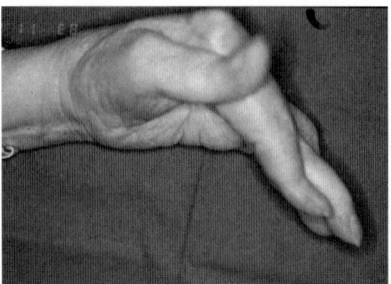

Fig. 3. Stiff fingers.

• Associated deformities due to bone and joint problems and ulnar drift allow an easy diagnosis.

1.2. Investigations

– Radiological images are grossly symmetrical for the two hands. There are no specific X-ray features for synovitis, except soft tissue swelling which may be visible on plain X-rays. Special views may demonstrate bone spikes, especially from the scaphoid bone. Bone erosions and cortex thinning are also typical of the disease.

Other examinations may help prior to medical or surgical treatment.

– MRI may demonstrate the extent and location of flexor tenosynovitis, especially when using gadolinium contrast enhancement. Tendon ruptures may also be seen, but this examination is not routinely used in this disease, as clinical and radiological examinations are usually sufficient. It may however be particularly useful at the beginning of the disease.
– High-frequency sonography is helpful in assessing even minimal finger tendon lesions in RA patients: thickening of flexor tendon sheath, loss of the normal fibrillar texture, nodules, irregularity of the flexor tendon, tendon tear. Complete or partial tendon rupture may be seen during flexion–extension movements, but this examination can be operator-dependent.

The severity of the disease and the degree of articular involvement in one particular patient is a better element of prognosis.

1.2.1. Literature review

– In one publication [3]: 188 tendons showed isolated synovitis, 208 had a tendon lesion with synovitis, 30 tendons showed a rupture. 81 showed tendon adhesions, 12 showed nodules, 63 showed superficial lesions and 52 defects were also detected. These lesions were found mainly in the palm of the second and third ray. Complaints and findings were different in the digit, palm, wrist and forearm.
– In another paper [4]: tenosynovitis of one or more flexor tendons of the hand was noted in 55% of 100 patients with rheumatoid arthritis (RA). The third flexor tendon was involved most frequently (71% of patients), followed by the second (62%), fourth

(53%), fifth (27%), and first (13%). Patients with flexor synovitis had a significantly higher prevalence of rheumatoid nodules (56% vs. 33%) and carpal tunnel syndrome (47% vs. 13%). Flexor carpi radialis and ulnaris synovitis were found exclusively in patients with flexor synovitis [5].

1.3. The thumb

There is also flexor pollicis longus synovitis and later a rupture of the same tendon: this rupture is secondary to tendon infiltration but also to attrition on a protruding scaphoid [6]. This rupture may be bilateral [7]. This bilateral rupture of the flexor pollicis longus was associated with subluxation and radial deviation of the carpus and increased angulation of the tendon in relation to the scaphoid.

2. Treatment

Medical treatment will be discussed elsewhere, as well as synoviortheses. With early and aggressive treatment involving new drug combinations, it may be possible to improve the course of RA and to prevent surgery in many cases.

Treatment has a significant effect on long-term results, but less on the evolution of the disease [8].

2.1. Treatment of nerve compression

1. Carpal tunnel syndrome (20% to 50% of the cases).
   It may be the first symptom of the disease. More proximal nerve compressions should be differentiated.
   A grading may be applied to indicate the treatment [9]: a) Mild synovitis may require conservative treatment only. b) Endoscopic carpal tunnel release, may be performed when moderate or quiescent synovitis is present [10]. Endoscopic release is contra-indicated if there is a synovitis with crepitus, loss of active finger flexion, if there is evidence of flexor tendon rupture or if surgery has been performed previously. c) Open carpal tunnel release combined with flexor tenosynovectomy is performed for severe synovitis. The nerve and its branches are released.
2. Guyon canal syndrome is rare and often associated with carpal tunnel syndrome. Bone destruction, hypertrophic synovitis or a synovial cyst may be a cause of compression. There may also be isolated or associated ulnar nerve compression at other sites.
   Decompression is performed in association with local treatments to the bone and joints.

2.2. Treatment of tenosynovitis

Early tenosynovectomy may prevent tendon ruptures and should therefore be the main treat-ment. It is combined with tendon realignment at the level of MP when an ulnar drift is present.

The Surgical Approach is undertaken through a longitudinal incision over the carpal tunnel, lazy S incision in the palm of the hand, and Bruner type over the volar aspect of the fingers.

(a) At the carpal tunnel, the median nerve is decompressed and mobilized (Fig. 4a, b). Synovectomy begins at this level. It allows tendon decompression and removes the synovitis which surrounds, invades and destroys the tendons. The tendon should lie in a

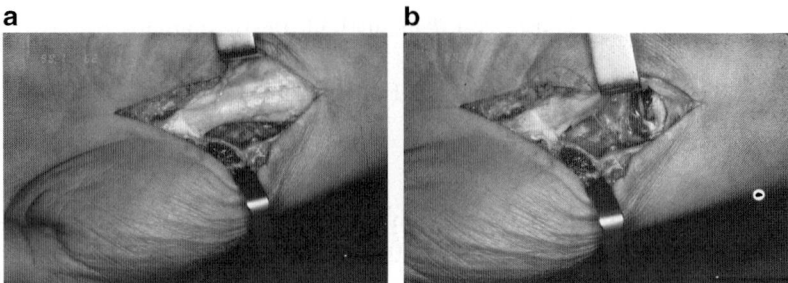

Fig. 4. Median nerve (a) decompressed and (b) mobilized.

decompressed area of healthy fat at the wrist and in the palm. The floor of the carpal tunnel is examined to look for bone spikes and spurs which may produce tendon tears and ruptures by attrition (Fig. 5). Removal of any bone spur is imperative in the treatment. Use of a flap of local capsule or flexor retinaculum to cover bone after osteophyte removal within the carpal tunnel [11] may also be indicated. All attrition ruptures occur within the carpal canal and represent the most common cause of tendon rupture.

Ruptures due to invasive tenosynovitis are frequently found within the carpal canal. These ruptures may be unanticipated, and may be discovered as an incidental finding during flexor tenosynovectomy.

(b) At the MP level: synovectomy is often combined with finger realignment. Cross intrinsic transfer can also be undertaken.

It is also possible to insert an implant or a prosthesis using the volar approach to realign destroyed joints. The deep transverse metacarpal ligament is cut three to four mm from the lateral border of the MP palmar plate. It is in anatomical continuity with the periosteum of the volar metacarpal and first phalanx and also with the MP volar plate. They are retracted "en bloc" and this allows an MP joint synovectomy to be undertaken. A prosthesis may then be inserted after bone preparation (Fig. 6). When closing, the transverse ligament is sutured with shortening and the distal and medial corner of the palmar plate is sutured to the collateral ligament of the MP joint.

(c) At the finger level, the fibrous canal has a fixed diameter and is not extensible. Flexor tenosynovitis should be treated with decompression and tenosynovectomy in the digital sheath and excision of the thickened synovium, not by incising the pulley

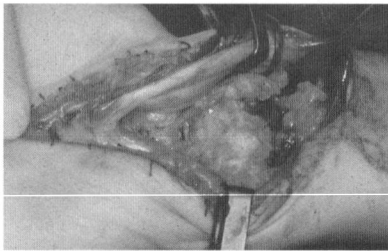

Fig. 5. Capsule tear and bone spike causing tendon rupture.

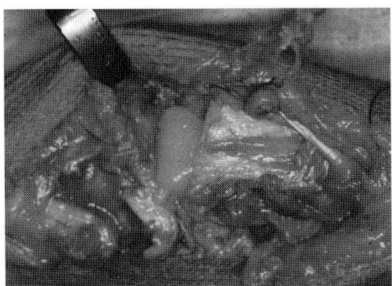

Fig. 6. Volar approach for inserting an MP prosthesis.

system. There is some controversy about resection of the proximal pulley (P1). There is a possibility without this pulley of accentuating the forces causing ulnar drift [12]. We have chosen an intermediate position resecting the pulley in an oblique way, keeping its ulnar wall. Some authors perform resection of the ulnar slip of the superficialis [13] in order to decompress the digital theca. Flexor synovectomy is not performed usually beyond the PIP joint. If the flexor profundus is impaired, a PID tenodesis is indicated.

Ruptures due to invasive tenosynovitis within the digit carry an unfavourable prognosis.

2.2.1. Literature review

– An analysis of the results of 201 hands operated on for flexor tendon synovectomy revealed that nearly 70% of the operated hands were subjectively improved; the others were unchanged or worse. The poor results were often caused by progression of the arthritis to finger joints. Recurrence of the tenosynovitis was observed in about 37% of the hands, but in very few to such an extent that reoperation had been necessary [14].
– Fifty patients were reviewed (64 hands) [15]: results obtained are reported at 4 months to eliminate any bias related to progression of the disease. The long-term results (follow-up: 8 years) are also analysed. Statistical analysis compares two groups depending on whether flexor tenosynovectomy was isolated (44%) or combined with a dorsal surgical procedure at the same operation (56%). Ninety percent of patients declared themselves to be subjectively improved. Objectively, mobility was always improved at 4 months then deteriorated to return to its preoperative level at 8 years. Only three patients were reoperated for recurrence. Flexor tenosynovectomy in rheumatoid arthritis is an excellent operation. Its analgesic effect is maintained in time and, when performed early, it appears to protect the patient from the risk of subsequent tendon rupture.
– 43 patients [16] who had rheumatoid arthritis of more than 15 years duration at the time of surgery were clinically assessed at a mean follow-up of 5.7 years (1.2–12 years). The patients had excellent sustained pain relief and were highly satisfied with the outcome of the procedure. 81% had adequate pulp-to-pulp and key pinch. Range of finger motion (total active motion, TAM) was excellent to good in 45% and fair in 22%. 33% were graded as poor and these were found to be multifactorial in origin, with

associated significant joint disease, preoperative tendon ruptures, extensive digital surgery, readhesions and combinations of operative procedures which adversely affect the rehabilitation programme. Flexor tenosynovectomy with tenolysis is a useful procedure with a low rate of recurrence.

– 235 operations on the flexor aspect of the hand performed on 139 patients are presented [17]. Results are very gratifying for tenosynovectomy in the carpal tunnel and pain. When performed on the fingers, however, 44% developed postoperative flexion contractures of various degrees, mainly when the synovectomy was extended beyond the level of the middle flexion crease of the finger.

– In a series [18] of nineteen hands (seventy-four fingers), there was restriction of active and passive motion of the proximal interphalangeal joints, with signs of flexor tenosynovitis but no clinical or roentgenographic evidence of involvement of the joint. The nineteen hands were treated by flexor tenosynovectomy (palm only in nine, palm and carpal tunnel in five, palm and digits in four, and digit, palm, and wrist in one) combined with manipulation of the joint under regional anesthesia. After an average follow-up of 21 months (range, 6 to 36 months), the average range of active motion had increased from 40° to 84° and the average range of passive motions, from 57° to 87°. Only three patients had unsatisfactory results, one because of persistent unexplained swelling and two because of recurrence of the tenosynovitis.

In conclusion, at an early stage, synovectomy of tendons gives good results with infrequent recurrence. It seems that it should not be performed beyond the PIP because the benefit is not proportional to the extent of surgery.

Surgical synovectomy is indicated when synovitis persists in spite of adequate medical treatment and should not be postponed for too long a period of time.

2.3. At the advanced stage

Flexor tenosynovectomy is combined with tendon repairs and prosthesis insertion. Improvement in flexion may also be obtained in 60% of the cases, depending on involvement of the dorsal tendons and the degree of bone and joint destruction at wrist and hand.

2.3.1. Tendon ruptures (Table 1)

The altered matrix of the tendon results in a weak tendon and rupture is the likely outcome after a variable evolution (Table 1). We believe that attrition on spurs is the main aetiology at the carpal tunnel level, but malposition of the carpus [19] (Fig. 7) and especially of the scaphoid is also a frequent cause. The volar ligament is thinned and torn in places. Sometimes, this follows a surgical procedure with metallic devices check.

Table 1
Digit involvement

III	71%
II	62%
IV	53%
V	27%
I	13%

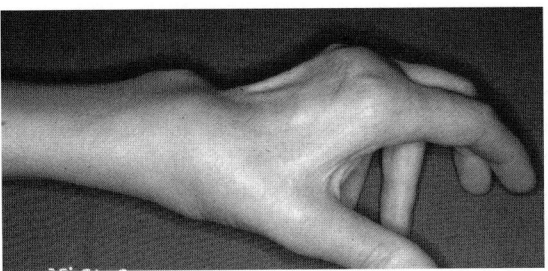

Fig. 7. Wrist malposition.

Tendon rupture and progressive adhesions to each other may mask the rupture. Sometimes tendon repairs are not mandatory when satisfactory movement is present.

(a) Repair is relatively easy for attrition ruptures by either suture, graft, overlapping or tendon transfer. If the profundus is ruptured, transfer of the superficialis to profundus or DIP arthrodesis is indicated. If the two tendons are ruptured, transfer the superficialis to the profundus.
(b) It is more difficult when synovial invasion of the tendon is diffuse and rupture is at different levels for the same tendon.

The prognosis for restoring flexion [7] in the event of a flexor tendon rupture is determined by the location of the rupture, aetiology, degree of articular involvement by the rheumatoid disease, and to a lesser degree, by the number of ruptured tendons. In general, isolated or double ruptures within the carpal canal due to attrition have a better prognosis than those caused by invasive tenosynovitis since the condition of the tendons is more favourable for reconstruction. As the number of ruptures increases, the prognosis in both conditions worsens. Rupture of both tendons within the digital sheath is quite difficult to treat, with ruptures in zone 2 carrying the worst prognosis for the restoration of flexion.

The severity of the patient's rheumatoid arthritis and articular disease has a great effect on the outcome of the reconstructive surgery. Prevention of tendon ruptures by early tenosynovectomy and the removal of bone spurs should be the goal of the surgeon.

Bone spikes may come from scaphoid, trapezium, triquetrum and lunate, hamatum, distal ulna and distal radius. They are due to bone and joint damages and to carpal destabilisation due to wrist ligament destructions, especially at the carpal first row.

Rupture frequency for the digits is reported in Table 2. Rupture at the digital level is far more serious.

Table 2
Flexor tendon ruptures (Nalebuff)

	Total	Attrition	Invasion
Wrist	91	61	30
Palm	4	0	4
Digits	20	0	20

2.3.2. Literature review

– Translocations of healthy tendons, overlapping to adjacent healthy tendons and tendon grafts were performed for 16 flexor tendons ruptures. For flexor tendons, there were 2 excellent results and 5 mediocre results in terms of thumb–palm contact. Prevention by early synovectomy is particularly important [20].
– 115 flexor tendon ruptures were reviewed in 45 hands with rheumatoid arthritis. 91 tendons were ruptured at the wrist, 4 ruptures occurred at the palm, and 20 ruptures occurred within the digits. At the wrist level, 61 ruptures were caused by attrition on a bone spur and 30 were caused by direct invasion of the tendon by tenosynovium. All ruptures distal to the wrist were caused by invasion of the tendon by tenosynovium. Patients whose ruptures were caused by attrition regained better motion than those whose ruptures were caused by invasion by tenosynovitis; however, overall motion was poor. Patients with isolated ruptures in the palm or at the wrist had the best functional results. Those patients with multiple ruptures within the carpal canal had a bad prognosis. Ruptures of both tendons within the fibro-osseous canal had the worst prognosis. The severity of the patient's disease and the degree of articular involvement had a great effect on the outcome of surgery. Prevention of tendon ruptures by early tenosynovectomy and removal of bone spurs should be the cornerstone of treatment [21].

3. Results

Results depend on wrist and finger joints status. Transfers obtain better results than grafts. The suture repair should be strong enough to allow early mobilization.

We should expect a motion of 20° (0–40) for flexion for the thumb and 55° (20–80) for a finger.

Rupture by attrition may achieve a flexion of 60% of normal and rupture by infiltration 40% of normal motion.

4. Conclusion

Volar involvement of flexor tendons is underestimated. Treatment should begin by flexor synovectomy which decreases finger desaxation. Rupture of one flexor tendon leads up to other tendon ruptures.

References

[1] E.M. Smith, et al., Flexor forces and rheumatoid metacarpophalangeal deformity, JAMA 198 (1966) 130–134.
[2] K.S. Wise, The anatomy of the metacarpo-phalangeal joints, with observations of the aetiology of ulnar drift, J. Bone Jt. Surg. 57B (1975) 485–490.
[3] A. Konig, G. Konig, Lesional pattern and clinical symptoms in rheumatoid flexor tendon disease, Z. Rheumatol. 58 (1999) 277–282.
[4] R.G. Gray, N.L. Gottlieb, Hand flexor tenosynovitis in rheumatoid arthritis. Prevalence, distribution, and associated rheumatic features, Arthritis Rheum. 20 (1977) 1003–1008.
[5] W. Grassi, et al., Finger tendon involvement in rheumatoid arthritis. Evaluation with high-frequency sonography, Arthritis Rheum. 38 (1995) 786–794.

 [6] L.G. Walker, Flexor pollicis longus rupture in rheumatoid arthritis secondary to attrition on a sesamoid, J. Hand Surg. 18A (1993) 990–991.
 [7] I. Spar, Flexor tendon ruptures in the rheumatoid hand: bilateral flexor pollicis longus rupture, Clin. Orthop. 127 (1977) 186–188.
 [8] B.R. Simmen, N. Gschwend, Tendon diseases in chronic rheumatoid arthritis, Orthopade 24 (1995) 224–233.
 [9] J. Shinoda, et al., Carpal tunnel syndrome grading system in rheumatoid arthritis, J. Orthop. Sci. 7 (2002) 188–193.
[10] H.J. Belcher, S. Varma, F. Schonauer, Endoscopic carpal tunnel release in selected rheumatoid patients, J. Hand Surg. 25 (2000) 451–452.
[11] P.J. Regan, et al., Use of a flap of flexor retinaculum to cover bone after osteophyte removal within the carpal tunnel, J. Hand Surg. 15B (1990) 109–110.
[12] D.C. Ferlic, M.L. Clayton, Synovectomy of the hand and wrist, Ann. Chir. Gynaecol. Suppl. 198 (1985) 26–30.
[13] D.C. Ferlic, M.L. Clayton, Flexor tenosynovectomy in the rheumatoid finger, J. Hand Surg. 3A (1978) 364–367.
[14] E. Dahl, O.A. Mikkelsen, J.U. Sorensen, Flexor tendon synovectomy of the hand in rheumatoid arthritis. A follow-up study of 201 operated hands, Scand. J. Rheumatol. 5 (1976) 103–107.
[15] R. Duche, et al., Tenosynovectomie des flechisseurs dans la polyarthrite rhumatoide. Etude analytique a court et a long terme de la mobilite des chaines digitales, Ann. Chir. Main Memb. Super. 12 (1993) 85–92.
[16] A.R. Tolat, J.K. Stanley, R.A. Evans, Flexor tenosynovectomy and tenolysis in longstanding rheumatoid arthritis, J. Hand Surg. 21 (1996) 538–543.
[17] O. Eiken, T. Haga, S. Salgeback, Volar tenosynovectomy in the rheumatoid hand, Scand. J. Plast. Reconstr. Surg. 10 (1976) 59–63.
[18] M.B. Millis, L.H. Millender, E.A. Nalebuff, Stiffness of the proximal interphalangeal joints in rheumatoid arthritis. The role of flexor tenosynovitis, J. Bone Jt. Surg. Am. 58 (1976) 801–805.
[19] J. Fourastier, Ruptures de tendons flechisseurs apres arthrodese partielle du carpe dans le poignet rhumatoide, Ann. Chir. Main Memb. Super. 14 (1995) 224–228.
[20] J.P. Aubert, et al., Les ruptures tendineuses a la main et au poignet dans la polyarth rite rhumatoide, J. Chir. 131 (1994) 420–422.
[21] A.N. Ertel, et al., Flexor tendon ruptures in patients with rheumatoid arthritis, J. Hand Surg. 13 (1988) 860–866.

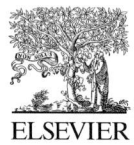

International Congress Series 1295 (2006) 118–128

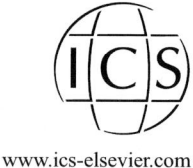

www.ics-elsevier.com

Surgery of the MCP joints in rheumatoid arthritis

F. Moutet *, D. Corcella, P. Pradel, A. Forli

Grenoble, France

Abstract. Two million people in Europe suffer with rheumatoid arthritis (RA). Among them 75% are women and the disease typically occurs around 45 years of age. Hand and wrist are almost always involved (over 80% of patients) and 70% of them will be obliged to stop their job. The ulnar drift of the metacarpophalangeal (MCP) joints is present in more than 36.5% of the cases in women. © 2006 Elsevier B.V. All rights reserved.

Keywords: Rheumatoid arthritis; Metacarpophalangeal joint

1. Introduction

Rheumatoid tenosynovitis has to be present to produce ulnar drift and there is no deformation at the MCP joint level without this tenosynovitis. When ténosynovites is present an average of 70% of the RA patients present with cartilage ulceration [1].

The deformation observed at the MCP of the long fingers joints is ulnar drift (Fig. 1). The reasons for this ulnar drift are many. Some are anatomical reasons: asymmetry of the metacarpal head, the longer length and the relative weakness (compared to the ulnar collateral ligament) of the radial collateral ligament. Other reasons include progression of the rheumatoid arthritis, tenosynovitis which weakens all the capsular system (lateral ligaments, volar plate and extensor hood), ulnar extensor apparatus dislocation and A1 pulley destruction. Some reasons are indirect consequences of the RA: ulnar gliding and radial drift of the carpus, abductor digiti minimi and intrinsic muscles contracture, lateral pinch of the thumb and grasp which push the long fingers to the ulnar border of the hand [2].

It must be emphasised that preventive surgery is the most effective treatment regarding MCP joint deformity. Actually wrist imbalance correction will protect the long fingers MCP joints from deformity for many years.

---

 * Corresponding author.
   E-mail address: Fmoutet@chu-grenoble.fr (F. Moutet).

0531-5131/ © 2006 Elsevier B.V. All rights reserved.
doi:10.1016/j.ics.2006.03.043

a   b

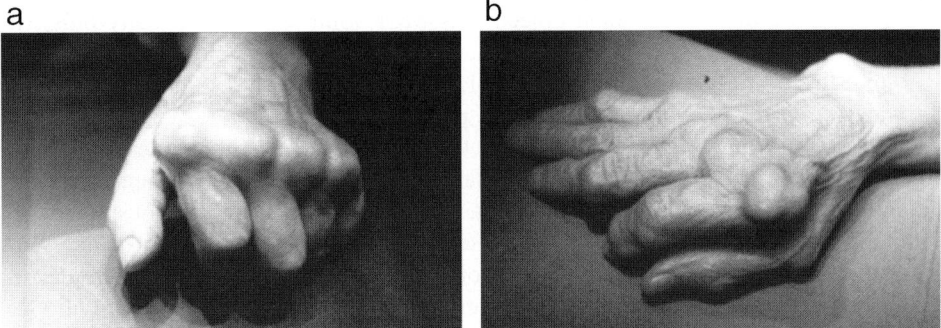

Fig. 1. Typical presentation of the ulnar drift in RA. (a) MCP joint dislocation is obvious and protrusion of the metacarpal head and sliding of the extensor apparatus in the ulnar intermetacarpal space. (b) Protrusive synovitis at the index and third finger MCP joint level can even mask an extensor tendon rupture.

As surgeons have for many years, rheumatologists now admit that their main objective regarding RA is to diagnose and treat as soon as possible. That means in the very first weeks or months after diagnosis. Actually the new medical treatments methotrexate (Methotrexate®, Novatrex®) and leflunomide (Arava®) have a clinical and structural efficiency by slowing down the evolution of the articular lesions [3]. So are the biotherapies anti-TNFα (Remicade®, Enbrel®, Humira®), or inhibitors of the action of the molecule interleukin-1 like Anakinra (Kineret®) or the monoclonal antibody anti CD20 Rituximab (Mabthera®).

2. Goals of surgery

The main goal of surgery is to prevent deformity whilst it is still possible. Unfortunately more often surgery is obliged to undertake palliative procedures (Fig. 2).

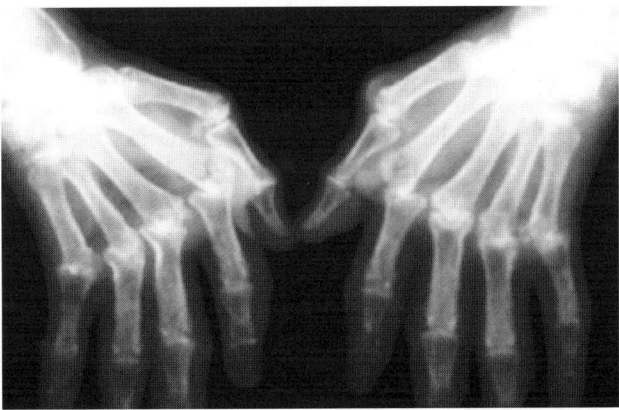

Fig. 2. Radiological final presentation of the hand at the MCP joints level. MCP joint of the thumb shows palmar dislocation with articular destruction. All the long fingers MCP joints are dislocated with articular destruction and ulnar drift.

Regarding the thumb, the main objective is MCP joint stability. Actually only MCP joint stability allows cylindrical grasp for handling a bottle or pen, etc. Easy to undertake, MCP joint fusion must be considered the gold standard for this type of surgery as it is the best way to improve the daily living of RA patients.

Regarding the long finger MCP joints, the problem is more complicated. Actually surgery must correct everything: the palmar dislocation, the extensor apparatus ulnar gliding and the imbalance of the whole joint. Tenosynovectomy, interosseous dorsal hood shortening and intrinsic muscles transfers attempt to correct this global imbalance. When articular destruction and palmar dislocation of the joint occur then arthroplasty is obviously indicated. For many years Swanson's silicone implant has been the gold standard in this field. Nowadays a new implant design with a more volar rotational axis and a more flexed resting position (30°) allows a great improvement in range of movement (ROM) especially in flexion and as a consequence a better grasp.

3. Strategy

The time honoured strategy advocated was always for sequential surgery. The wrist had to be operated first, followed by MCP joints and then the thumb. However, this may not be the best way. Actually too numerous successive procedures are discouraging for patients. One has to remember that not only are the hand and wrist involved but also very often other small or big joints which may require surgery. For that reason it would seem sensible to gather several surgical procedures to the hand and wrist together. That means that the wrist, long fingers MCP joints and the MCP of the thumb must be included in the same surgical procedure if appropriate.

4. The surgical challenge

4.1. Regarding the MCP of the thumb

As said before regarding the MCP joint of the thumb the main goal of surgery is to obtain a stable strong and opposable thumb. No prosthesis can ensure a lateral stability safe enough to assume the amount of strength required for lateral pinch. As a consequence the golden standard regarding the MCP joint of the thumb remains fusion of the joint. It is a very valuable surgical procedure, easy, safe and reliable. It may be undertaken as an out-patient and can prove to undecided patients the role of surgical treatment. It is the perfect example of a "winner procedure" that you may propose when you are looking to convince the patient and sometimes the rheumatologist of the benefits of the whole surgical program.

Whatever the surgical technique is, the average time for clinical and radiographic fusion is between 6 to 8 weeks [4].

4.2. Regarding the MCP of the long fingers

The principle cause of all MCP joint dislocation is the radial drift of the carpal bones due to the distal radio-ulnar joint dislocation followed by the medial ECU gliding permitting its loosening. This allows the extensor apparatus to dislocate into the ulnar intermetacarpal space and its "bow-stringing" on the ulnar side of the MCP joints.

Associated with the laxity of all the articular capsule components, this tension allows the ulnar drift to occur.

With regard to the treatment of the long finger MCP joints, obviously fusion is unacceptable and only a procedure allowing useful movement conservation must be done. Before any decision regarding surgical procedure is taken however, one must answer the question: Are the articular surfaces preserved? If the answer is yes the second question is: Are the soft tissues around the joint available or not for a surgical reconstructive procedure? If the answer is yes, then conservative treatment may be appropriate. If the answer is no to one or both of these questions, then two options may be discussed: The first one is the arthroplastic or prosthetic replacement of the joint; the other is fusion of the joint. At the long fingers MCP joint level, this last solution is inappropriate as discussed previously.

5. Options

5.1. Tenosynovectomy

When tenosynovitis is isolated to a particular joint, pain and functional impairment are the principal symptoms. If local steroid injections or the new medical treatments fail to reduce tenosynovitis, surgical tenosynovectomy may be undertaken.

Surgical removal or destruction of the diseased synovium is a more rational method of treatment. Of course it would be a more valuable procedure when done as a preventive measure before secondary changes have occurred in the joints. But one must be careful because the joints do not always react favourably to surgical intervention and some restriction in the range of movement may follow tenosynovectomy. Patients must be warned of this stiffness because most of them tend to expect immediate and miraculous benefits from the operation. It must be clear that the object of the operation is not the cosmetic improvement of the swollen joint but the prevention in the future of more drastic troubles by removing the primary site of the disease as described by Flatt many years ago [5].

In any event tenosynovectomy remains the first step of any surgical undertaking to the MCP joints of the long fingers. Usually there is a large dorsal and proximal pouch of synovium that must be stripped up from the neck and head of the metacarpal before the true joint cavity is entered. Pituitary rongeurs are a very useful instrument for removing the tongue of synovium that lies between the collateral ligament and the side of the metacarpal head. Tenosynovectomy can only be done in isolation if the cartilage and articular surfaces are good enough to allow full passive range of movement (ROM). Then tenosynovectomy is a worthwhile procedure. It diminishes pain, conserves or improves function and delays local RA evolution. It doesn't however prevent further recurrences, which depend on the efficacy of the medical treatment.

Very often the skin of the RA patients is thin and fragile. This cause of a potential local complication must be kept in mind for any kind of procedure. Gentle dissection is the best way to avoid skin necrosis and so infection. The skin incision must be chosen as a part of a whole therapeutic strategy. That means that one must always think about potential future interventions. As a consequence we strongly recommend a slightly curved incision to the ulnar side of the MCP for the 2nd and 4th finger MCP and radial side of the 3rd and 5th. So if a future procedure is needed these incisions are able to be included in "Y" shaped incisions with minimal consequences.

5.2. Soft tissue reconstruction

One must not forget that soft tissue reconstructions are temporary treatments. In the course of time their benefits will inevitably diminish. They must not be done if the articular surfaces of the joints are destroyed or if the palmar dislocation is not easily reducible.

The gold standard of soft tissue reconstruction is still dorsal hood shortening but as has been said before the hood has to be strong enough for it to be of value. Many techniques are being used (Fig. 3) [6].

At surgery one must pay special attention to the reconstruction of the radial collateral ligament (RCL). The best way to do this is to detach the elongated radial collateral ligament near its origin after tenosynovectomy of the dorsal aspect of the MCP. After detachment of the RCL the palmar aspect of the joint can be cleared easily. Then the ligament is shortened and reinserted dorsally to gain slight supination [7].

Use of the volar plate for reconstructing the radial collateral ligament after MCP joint tenosynovectomy may also be recommended either for soft tissue reconstruction alone or after arthroplasty [8]. Actually the volar plate is often intact and may be used for several purposes; reconstructing the RCL or as an interposition arthroplasty as described by Tupper.

Very often there is no clinical correlation between the active range of motion, synovitis or X-rays. Results may be stable for many years. Any soft tissue reconstruction associated with tenosynovectomy should be done as soon as possible. It affords protection of the joint during the early years before there is a requirement for arthroplasty.

5.3. MCP joints arthroplasty

Before any procedure of this type is undertaken, one must verify if the extensor and flexor tendons are strong enough to mobilize a reconstructed joint. If they are not, a prior or simultaneous reconstruction of the tendons must be undertaken. Proximal interphalangeal (PIP) joint function has to be examined also. Actually the final functional result depends on all these associated tendinous and articular factors.

5.3.1. Autologous arthroplasty

Following Bunnell who advocated metacarpal head resection, a lot of procedures have been proposed. They all interpose a soft tissue structure into the space between the bones. Only the Tupper's method which uses the volar plate as an interposition material seems to be satisfactory [9]. All the other materials (perichondrium, free articular toe transfer, etc.) have been abandoned. These types of procedures often lead to osseous resorption and recurrence of the deformity. Furthermore, the structures you need to undertake at surgery are not always found in sufficient quality or quantity. As a consequence indications are very few.

5.3.2. Metallic arthroplasty

Nowadays there is no place for the metallic hinge prosthesis in RA as proposed 30 or 40 years ago. Even with the sophisticated hinge prosthesis the residual bone stock and the stress transfer are a cause of loosening, dislocation or rupture of the prosthesis, even metacarpal or phalangeal shaft fractures.

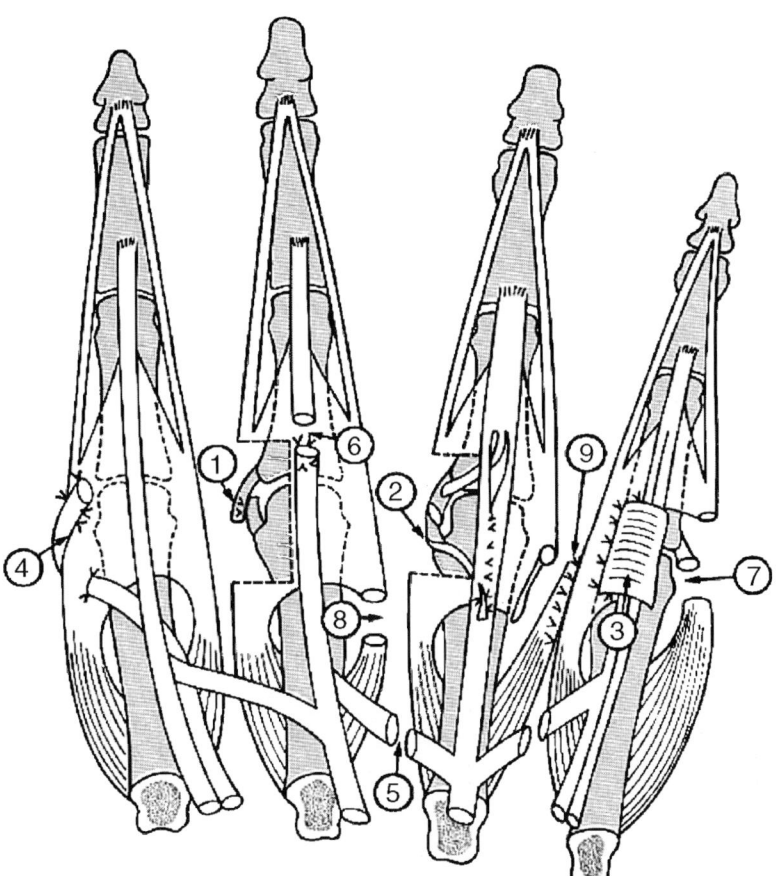

Fig. 3. Main surgical techniques for soft tissue reconstruction [6].

Using capsule and ligaments

1- Shorhortening of the RCL
2- RCL reinforcement

Using extensor apparatus

3- Dorsal hood covering suture
4- Extensor indicis proprius transfer
5- Junctura tendinorum resection
6- Extensor Ccmmunis dorsal reinsertion at the base of the proximal phalanx

Using interosseous muscles

7- Abductor digiti minimi tendon section
8- Ulnar intrinsic muscles section
9- Intrinsic muscles transfer

5.3.3. Silicone implant

5.3.3.1. Surgical procedure.   An approach to the MCP joints may be undertaken through a lazy S transversal incision on the dorsal aspect of the four MCP joints. This standard approach is however under tension while rehabilitating flexion, even under a protective splint. As a consequence we now prefer a "Y" shaped incision which is repeated over the dorsal aspect of the second and fourth web space if needed. This gives an excellent exposure of the four MCP joints and is safer regarding skin tension during mobilization. Furthermore it may include an earlier skin incision used for isolated tenosynovectomy as stated previously (Fig. 4).

The dorsal hood of the extensor apparatus is released on its radial aspect. If its appearance is satisfactory it will allow reconstruction by pulling back the extensor tendon over the dorsum of the MP joint using a suture. If it is obviously not possible, one may only divide the hood on its ulnar aspect and leave it open.

As usual tenosynovectomy is the first step of the procedure. Then the metacarpal head is cut with an electric saw close but distal to the insertion of the collateral ligament of the MCP joint or after its detachment. These ligaments are kept intact as far as possible. The oblique section of the metacarpal must be a little more radial that the anatomical plane of the MCP joint. This is the main factor for rebalancing the MCP joints. Originally Swanson's technique asked us not to touch the bone of the proximal phalanx. Actually it is

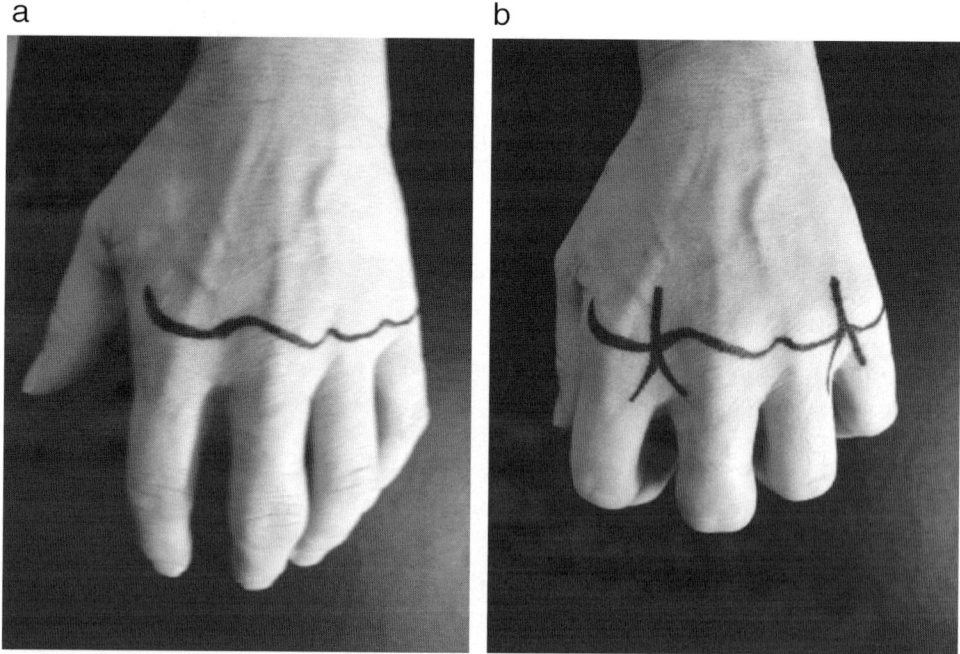

Fig. 4. Skin incision. (a) Usual lazy "S" quite transversal skin incision. (b) "Y" shaped incisions compared to the lazy "S". "Y" shaped one allows less tension while moving the MCP joints. Any part of the "Y" may be use in a first procedure and then used for other procedures.

useful to resect this surface especially to make the metacarpal and the phalangeal surfaces as parallel as possible according to the new flexion plane which is more radial than before. In addition this also protects the implant surfaces from sharp bone edges which can result in implant fracture [10].

The volar plate may be excised allowing a better ROM or detached to be used for RCL reconstruction as described. In any event soft-tissue reconstruction is usually advocated as an adjunct to MCP joint arthroplasty. RCL reconstruction jointly with abductor digiti mini release at the fifth MCP joint restores the balance of forces around the MCP joint but can't prevent late postoperative deformity. Actually recurrence is a common problem as in all the isolated soft-tissue reconstruction [11].

We believe, as do more and more authors, that the most worthwhile procedure to obtain good and permanent correction of the ulnar drift after arthroplasty of the MCP joint is not the soft tissue reconstruction. We think that the appropriate bone resection combined with good quality capsular healing around the silicone implant (synovialization) facilitated by dynamic splinting for a long period (between 6 and 8 weeks) post operatively are the two main factors of success.

5.3.3.2. Implant choice.   The "gold standard" for many years has been the silicone implant proposed by Swanson [12]. However, long-term follow-up reveals an increasing number of complications particularly mechanical failures.

After Swanson's arthroplasty the mean arc of motion often improves from 40° to 60° although this outcome often worsens with long term follow-up [13]. Trail et al reported that after a long time period (over 17 years), two-thirds of the implants were seen to be broken and the use of grommets did not protect the implant from fracture. Soft tissue-balancing, crossed intrinsic transfer and realignment of the wrist are factors that improved the survival of the implants [14].

In order to deal with these problems a number of new, biomechanically different silicone implants have been designed. Among these we prefer the Neuflex® prosthesis (Fig. 5). It has a preflexed hinge of 30° in relation to the shaft axis (corresponding to the normal resting position of the hand), a more palmar lying center of rotation (which reduces

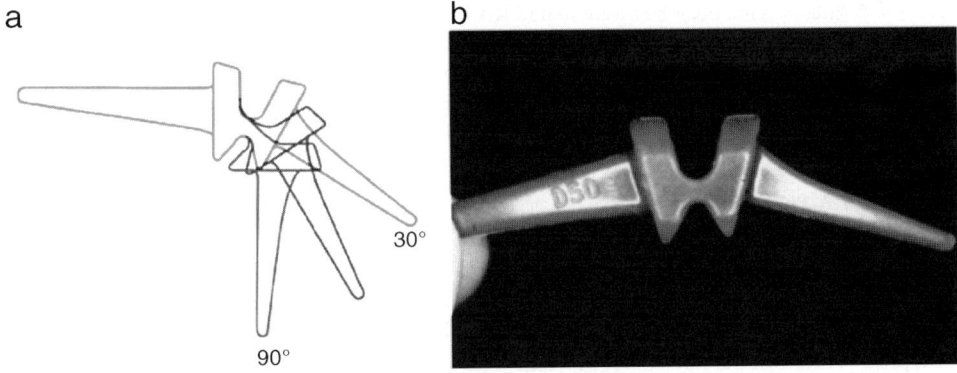

Fig. 5. Neuflex® implant. (a) Design and ROM of the implant. (b) One can notice the preflexed position of 30° corresponding to the normal resting position of the MCP joints.

strain across the hinge by 35%) and a rectangular hinge with a collar like platform abutting the bony surfaces. The advantage of this new design is an improved overall range of movement in the MCP joint with better grip function. The improved flexor tendon excursion and moment arm appear to be the main reasons for the substantially improved flexion following the use of the Neuflex® device. This implant improves a little bit the extensor lag but significantly improves flexion by around 15° when compared to the Swanson implants [15]. Overall the Neuflex® silicone implants show encouraging early results which must now be confirmed in the long term.

Whatever the implant is, the metacarpal and phalangeal shafts have to be prepared very gently with the appropriate rasps. Swanson and many authors after him recommended that as big an implant as possible is used. It may be better however to use the safest one. That means not to jeopardize the bone stock especially at the phalangeal level, try to keep the lateral ligaments intact and restore a convenient tension of the joint. Stabilization of the implant may be undertaken accordingly with all the soft tissue reconstruction techniques available. In any event it is the bone resection which is the most important part of the technique and will assure the implant stability. One should not think that soft tissue reconstruction alone will confer implant stability.

The surface replacement implants made of pyrocarbon may become an alternative to silicone spacers although at this time there is insufficient follow up [16].

5.3.3.3. Complications. As has been stated previously silicone implants have a number of complications. Some are mechanical failures, either fractures, or dislocation. Some are due to the biomechanical environment as the stems piston in the bone shafts causing bone resorption and hyperostosis. Some are biological due to silicone fragmentation. This severe complication is due to a foreign body reaction related to silicone microparticles. It is a rare complication despite the fact that MCP joint implants are stressed in flexion. It is more a complication of implants working in compression like the scaphoid, lunate or even trapezium implants. Furthermore implant fracture does not always require implant removal and if it does a simple implant exchange is often sufficient.

5.3.3.4. Results. One must be aware that in RA it is not always clear what determines satisfaction with MCP joint replacement surgery. The surgeon focuses primarily on objective outcomes such as ROM or strength. The strongest determinant of patient satisfaction seems to be postoperative hand appearance and pain decrease. Ability to perform activities of daily living, hand strength and ROM show minimal correlation with patients' overall satisfaction [17].

6. Postoperative cares

6.1. Goals of rehabilitation

Rehabilitation, physical and occupational therapy together is a whole part of the treatment. Nothing can be done and nothing will work without it. Splinting is one of the numerous components of a complete treatment. After the dynamic splinting for correction of the ulnar drift, rest splints must always be worn by the patient nightly and indefinitely.

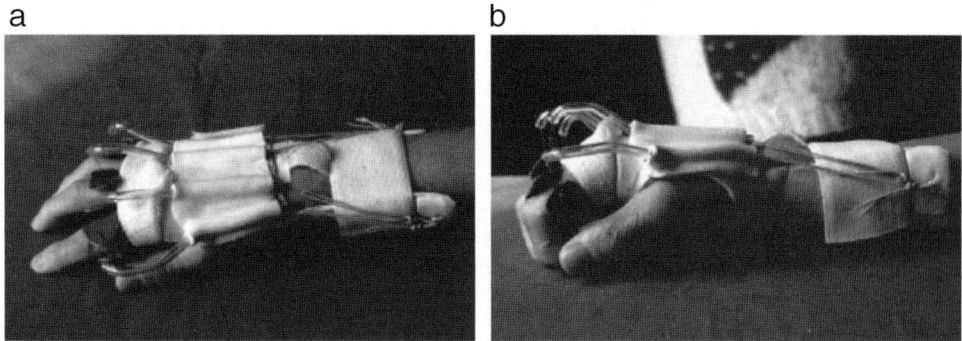

Fig. 6. Postoperative splinting. (a) Low profile splint with radial traction protecting the soft tissue reconstruction with or without MCP joints implants. (b) The splint allows active flexion of the MCP joints from 0° to 45° protected by dorsal traction.

6.2. Goals of splinting

As has been stated previously splinting is an important part of the postoperative treatment and it is especially true regarding MCP joints surgery in RA. Dynamic splinting will protect the extensor balance and surgical reconstruction. It must allow light active MCP joint flexion around 40–45° (Fig. 6). After 6 weeks the dynamic splintage may be stopped and daily activities restored. Only the rest splint is used every night.

In all cases total collaboration must be instigated between the surgeon, the therapists and the rheumatologist to accord the appropriate medical treatment given the progression of the disease and the patient needs.

Whatever the surgical procedure is, surgery is only a part of the whole treatment. Furthermore not only rehabilitation but also education must be undertaken. An educational program for RA is worthwhile and has to be a part of the global treatment. The patient must have as clear as possible an idea of what he safely can do and what he can't during his daily living.

7. Conclusion

One must keep in mind the incredible adaptive capacities of RA patients. Hand function is undoubtedly severely impaired by the ulnar drift and palmar dislocation of the MCP joint. However, physicians must be attentive to the patient's complaints. Discussions about surgical intervention in the severely deformed hand must be tempered in the absence of pain and some preserved function.

Surgical management of the rheumatoid hand is still the subject of controversy among rheumatologists and hand surgeons. In 2003 a study from the US showed that 70% of rheumatologists consider hand surgeons deficient in understanding the medical options available, while 73.6% of surgeons believe rheumatologists have insufficient knowledge of the surgical options. [18]. It is therefore obviously necessary to focus on improving communication between rheumatologists and hand surgeons to improve patient benefit.

It is clear for us that, whatever the surgical procedure was, is or will be, a multidisciplinary approach is the only way to give to the patient the best care he or she deserves. That means a global strategy accepted by all the members of the therapeutical team of which the patient is first [19].

References

[1] V.A.I. Laine, E. Sairanen, K.J. Vainio, Fingers deformities caused by rheumatoid arthritis, J. Bone Jt. Surg. 39A (1957) 527.

[2] D.V. Egloff, La main et le poignet rhumatoïde traitement chirurgical, in: Y. Allieu (Ed.), Monographie du GEM N°23 Expansion Scientifique Française Paris, 1996, pp. 105–120.

[3] D. Van Der Heidje, et al., Presentation and analysis of data on radiographic outcome in clinical trials: experience of the TEMPO study, Arthritis Rheum. 52 (2005) 49–60.

[4] C.C. Schmidt, S.M. Zimmer, S.D. Boles, Arthrodesis of the thumb metacarpophalangeal joint using a cannulated screw and threaded washer, J. Hand Surg. (Am.) 29 (6) (2004) 1044–1050.

[5] A.E. Flatt, The Care of the Arthritic Hand, 5th edition, Quality Medical Publishing, St. Louis, 1995, pp. 268–319.

[6] Y. Allieu, B. Brahin, Les déformations de la main rhumatoïde et leurs traitements, Documenta Geigy, 1985, pp. 55–71.

[7] K. Das Gupta, P. Haussman, Synovialectomy of the metacarpophalangeal joints with reconstruction of the radial collateral ligaments—long-term results in patients suffering from rheumatoid arthritis, Hanchir. Mikrochir. Plast. Chir. 37 (1) (2005) 35–39.

[8] H.E. Kleinert, T.M. Sunil, Use of volar plate for reconstructing the radial collateral ligament after metacarpophalangeal arthroplasty of fingers in rheumatoid arthritis: surgical technique, J. Hand Surg. (Am.) 30 (2) (2005) 390–393.

[9] J.M. Tupper, The volar plate arthroplasty for rheumatoid arthritis. Its rationale and technique, Sekei. Geka 23 (1972) 1137–1140.

[10] I. Mannerfelt, K. Andersson, Silastic arthroplasty of the metacarpophalangeal joints in rheumatoid arthritis. Long term results, J. Bone Jt. Surg. 57A (1975) 484–489.

[11] H. Burezq, et al., The value of radial collateral ligament reconstruction and abductor digiti minimi release in metacarpophalangeal joint arthroplasty, Ann. Plast. Surg. 54 (4) (2005) 397–401.

[12] A.B. Swanson, Flexible implant arthroplasty for arthritic finger joint, J. Bone Jt. Surg. (1972) 435–455.

[13] C.A. Goldfarb, P.J. Stern, Metacarpophalangeal joint arthroplasty in rheumatoid arthritis. A long-term assessment, J. Bone Jt. Surg., Am. 86-A (8) (2004) 1832–1833.

[14] I.A. Trail, et al., Seventeen-year survivorship analysis of silastic metacarpophalangeal joint replacement, J. Bone Jt. Surg., Br. 86 (7) (2004) 1002–1006.

[15] R. Delaney, I.A. Trail, D. Nuttall, A comparative study of outcome between the Neuflex and Swanson metacarpophalangeal joint replacements, J. Bone Jt. Surg., Br. 30 (1) (2005) 3–7.

[16] R.D. Beckenbaugh, Arthroplasty of the metacarpophalangeal joint using pyrocarbonate implants, Orthopade 32 (9) (2003) 794–797.

[17] L.A. Mandl, et al., Metacarpophalangeal arthroplasty in rheumatoid arthritis: what determines satisfaction with surgery? J. Rheumatol. 29 (12) (2002) 2477–2483.

[18] A.K. Alderman, et al., Surgical management of the rheumatoid hand: consensus and controversy among rheumatologists and hand surgeons, J. Rheumatol. 30 (7) (2003) 1464–1472.

[19] H.M. Kremers, et al., Therapeutic strategies in rheumatoid arthritis over a 40-year period, J. Rheumatol. 31 (2004) 2366–2373.

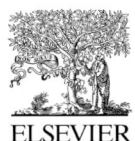
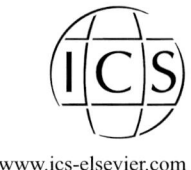
Silastic metacarpophalangeal joint arthroplasty

I.A. Trail *

Hand and Upper Limb Surgery, Wrightington, Wigan and Leigh NHS Trust, Hall Lane, Appley Bridge, Wigan, Lancs, WN6 9EP, England, United Kingdom

Abstract. Of all the joints of the hand arthroplasty of the metacarpophalangeal joint of the fingers has been most widely undertaken and probably the most successful procedure. The success is in no small matter due to the success of silicone hinged implants at this site, combined with this joints frequent involvement in patients with rheumatoid arthritis. As a consequence the replacement of this joint in this group of patients has become the operation of choice, with long term benefits reported over many years. In 1968 Swanson and Niebauer reported the use of a silicone rubber spacer metacarpophalangeal joint replacement (Fig. 1). At that time they reported good to excellent short term results, which have ultimately been reproduced throughout the world. From that time there have been a number of further developments of this type of implant with an improvement in the materials used, and also the design. The use of this type of silicone-based implant has been so successful that it is now hard to envisage that any hand surgery unit does not use this type of implant on a routine basis. As stated previously the indication par excellence for arthroplasty of the metacarpophalangeal joint is inflammatory arthritis, particularly rheumatoid arthritis and it is in this situation that the hinged silastic implant has been proved to be ideal. For other indications however, particularly trauma or osteoarthritis, silastic has been less successful, the principal reason being that in the otherwise normal hand the forces applied to the implant quite quickly result in failure of the silastic. As a consequence of this newer two-part prosthesis has been developed that is often made of titanium or cobalt chrome with high density polyethylene, the designs often mimicking normal anatomy. More recently a newer material, pyro-carbon, has become available. With these new implants, however, have come changes in surgical technique. For the silastic implants essentially the procedure is one of an excision arthroplasty with the silastic acting as an internal splint, allowing the soft tissues to rebalance. Plainly this is not the case with the two-part implants and as such greater care has to be taken with regard to bone resection and realignment as instability can be a significant problem. © 2006 Published by Elsevier B.V.

Keywords: Metacarpophalangeal joint arthroplasty; Silicone implant; Swanson implant

---

* Tel.: +44 1257 256248.
  E-mail address: upperlimb@wrightington.org.uk.

0531-5131/ © 2006 Published by Elsevier B.V.
doi:10.1016/j.ics.2006.03.01

1. Surgical technique

Silastic metacarpophalangeal joint replacement has been undertaken by surgeons throughout the world for a number of years. The surgical procedure was first described concurrently by Swanson and Niebauer in the 1970s (Fig. 1). Usually the operation is undertaken either under full general anaesthesia or a complete regional block with sedation. The patient lies in a supine position with a tourniquet in place. At this time it is important to remember that if the procedure is undertaken under regional anaesthesia the pressure of the tourniquet can cause more concern to the patient than the procedure more distally. With regard to the procedure itself however, it is important to emphasise that first and foremost this is an excision arthroplasty with realignment. The latter being undertaken by a sequence of releases and reconstruction of tendons and ligaments. The silastic implant acts merely as a flexible spacer, allowing earlier mobilization with the finger in the corrected position. As a consequence management of the soft tissues surrounding the metacarpophalangeal joint is of paramount importance. Indeed many would say that this is more important than the actual insertion of the silastic implant.

For the skin incision either a transverse incision or longitudinal incision lying directly over the metacarpophalangeal joint or in the gullies between them can be employed. Certainly the exposure of the individual joint is better with a longitudinal incision. A transverse incision however allows all the joints to be exposed through one incision which gives better long term cosmesis. It is important however that if a transverse incision is used this does not lie directly over the metacarpophalangeal joint but more proximally over the metacarpal head. The incision will also have to be extended down the radial side of the index finger and ulna side of the little finger joint. When the skin incision is made it is important to preserve as many of the subcutaneous vessels and nerves as possible. Ideally these can be displaced into the gullies between the joints. The extensor hood is then identified. In the vast majority of cases of rheumatoid arthritis the extensor tendon has displaced in an ulnar direction and can often lie in the gulley itself. This must be released on both the radial and ulnar sides so that at the end of the procedure it can be repositioned

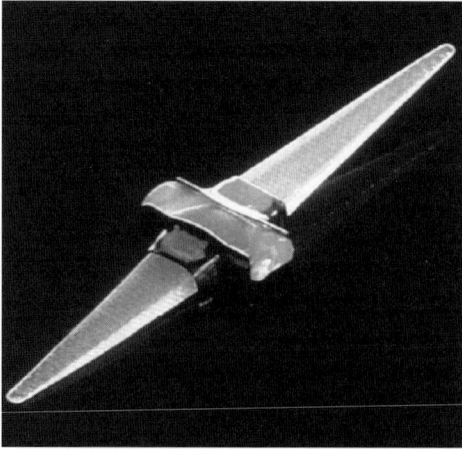

Fig. 1. Swanson silicone metacarpophalangeal joint arthroplasty.

over the apex of the joint. This release will also allow the joint itself to be exposed. The capsule of the joint is then identified and incised longitudinally. It is important to remember that in many cases of advanced rheumatoid arthritis the capsule can be thin and adherent to the under surface of the extensor tendon and as such may not be a distinct structure.

The articular surfaces are then visualised and the clinical and radiological appearances are confirmed. Joint replacement should only then be undertaken if the articular surfaces are significantly involved in the disease process. Otherwise synovectomy with soft tissue realignment is all that is needed. As to the technique for removal of the articular surface, the reader is referred to the relevant manufacturers' operative instructions. However, as this is an excision arthroplasty the whole of the metacarpal head can be removed as well as a sliver of the base of the proximal phalanx. With regard to the proximal phalanx as the joint could well have been subluxed for some time, erosion of the articular surface particularly superiorly is not uncommon. However, it is essential that whatever prosthesis is used the cuts are perpendicular and no sharp edges are left to impinge on the silastic replacement.

At this stage the collateral ligaments and intrinsics can be addressed. Essentially all structures on the ulnar side can be released from either the metacarpal or proximal phalanx. This would involve particularly the ulnar collateral ligament and volar plate. On the radial side if the joint is particularly tight then again the collateral can be released, although generally it is preferable to retain this structure or if it is lax shorten to tighten the radial side. For the index finger traditionally the radial collateral ligament is released off the metacarpal and reattached proximally and dorsally. This has the effect of pronating the finger and aiding pinch. On the volar aspect of the joint the volar plate can often be contracted as a result of a long standing flexion deformity indeed volar subluxation of the metacarpophalangeal joint. Again this structure will have to be released from the proximal phalanx.

At this point it is better to prepare to insert the trial prosthesis and assess movement and stability. As stated previously the method of resecting bone can vary between manufacturers. In general however it is vital that enough bone is removed to allow the implant to be freely seated. The intramedullary canals of the metacarpal and proximal phalanx are prepared again as per the manufacturers' recommendation. Once the trial has been inserted a true assessment of stability and alignment can be undertaken. This was first appreciated by Swanson who noted that if there was a continuing deformity this would result in subluxation of the implant and if the space was too tight this would result in compression of the implant and reduced movement. (Fig. 2).

Finally and more recently soft tissue rebalancing has been supplemented by a crossed intrinsic transfer. Traditionally the intrinsics were released particularly if they caused a contracture. The latter would be demonstrated by placing the MCP joints in extension and passively flexing the proximal interphalangeal joint. Intrinsic tightening would prevent this from occurring. Cross intrinsic transfer however takes the divided intrinsic on the ulnar side of the digit and inserts it into the collateral ligament on the radial side of the adjacent digit (Fig. 3). The rationale being this will prevent subsequent ulnar deviation. Obviously this procedure can only be undertaken for the middle, ring and little fingers.

Joint Relationship And Spacer Concept

SUBLUXED   TOO TIGHT   CORRECT

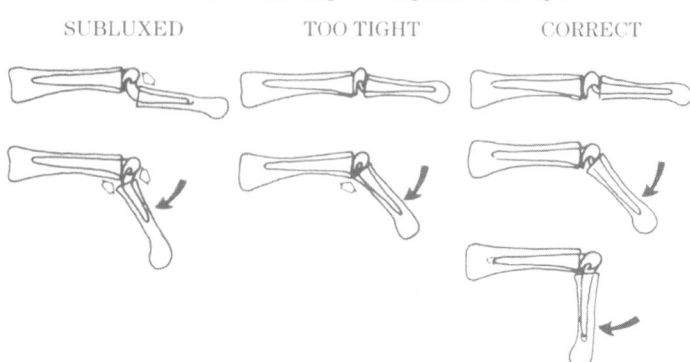

Fig. 2. Balance across the MCP joint.

Once the true implant is in situ the capsule can be repaired and closed. It is however crucial to realign the extensor tendon directly over the metacarpophalangeal joint. This is undertaken by suturing the tendon down into the midline. While this obviously will reduce any excursion of the tendon it should be remembered that the extensor tendon acts predominantly at the metacarpophalangeal joint. The skin is then sutured and a drain left in situ. We remove the drain at 48h and the sutures at between 10 and 14 days.

2. Rehabilitation

The following is a description of a therapy protocol currently used at Wrightington Hospital. I am obviously therefore indebted to all the therapists at Wrightington for their help and of course allowing me to present their treatment protocols. I am also aware that many different regimes are in use at hand centres throughout the world. Plainly however it would be outside the remit of this publication to present all the different variations in therapy.

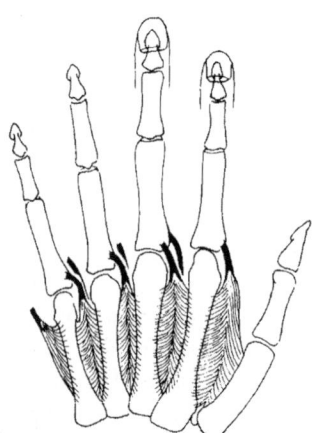

Fig. 3. Cross intrinsic transfer.

Following surgery the patients arm is elevated to prevent swelling and the neurovascular status of the fingers are monitored. At the same time it is important to provide the patient with adequate analgesia. This can take the form of an infusion of narcotic as required or some form of proximal nerve block. On day two the immediate postoperative dressings are removed and the wound is inspected; at that time any drains are also removed. The wound is redressed and if satisfactory a plaster of Paris slab is applied to the volar side. If this is not possible then a resting splint can be manufactured.

Between days three and five the patient continues to elevate the hand and receive appropriate pain relief. On day five an outrigger (Fig. 4) is constructed and an exercise regime instigated. At the same time the patient is given instruction with regard to the activities of daily living. Ideally this should be done prior to discharge.

On day fourteen the sutures are removed. At that time and up to 6 weeks following surgery the patient continues with the outrigger during the day and the resting splint at night; exercises are ongoing. In addition to that scar massage may be undertaken. Static flexion and extension splints are also manufactured if appropriate.

From 6 weeks the outrigger is discarded, while the night splintage continues, the latter for a further 6 weeks. During this period however, light function can be gained while joint protection advice is given. The latter involves performing activities of daily living (ADL) through a directed active exercise programme. This allows muscle strength to improve as well as increasing the range of movement of the joints. It is however important to avoid external forces on joints, particularly those that will produce ulnar deviation. Simply this would include building up handles on objects and substitute gross grasp or tripod pinch for lateral pinch. An appropriate ulnar deviation splint could also be utilised.

Thirdly, alterations in normal day to day activities help, for example, carrying a tray on the forearm making use of multiple joints to undertake the activity. Another simple change would involve changing a hand bag for a shoulder bag. At the same time avoid using the MCP joints to apply force. If crutches are required, forearm crutches would be preferable. In addition it is often sensible to recommend to the patient that they adopt a good posture and make full use of the intrinsic/extrinsic muscle groups to prevent imbalance. An example of this would be to flex the fingers by flexing the small joints first before the metacarpophalangeals and extending the metacarpophalangeals before the smaller joints.

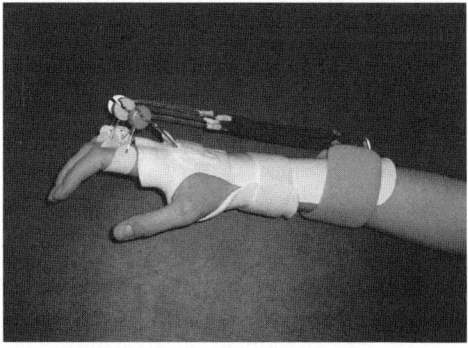

Fig. 4. Typical dynamic outrigger.

Finally, any sustained activity will often cause muscle fatigue, ligamentous strain, but also ultimately could damage the arthroplasty. The answer to this is to balance the activity with rest, in other words undertake activity for less time but more frequently. In light of this it is also important to avoid activities that cannot be immediately halted. At work again appropriate time and motion activities will protect the joint. It is also important that patients are taught to respect pain. Any pain and discomfort that persists for several hours after a task is most certainly not beneficial.

While the above treatment regime is probably the most widely used many variations are in common use. Indeed a number of departments have questioned the value of dynamic splintage.

At this time unfortunately there is little in the way of any good prospective study to confirm the value of an extensor splint or indeed any of the alternatives. This was confirmed by Massy-Westrop and Krishnan [14] from Australia, who concluded after a literature search that the main differences between the various postoperative regimes was the use of passive MCP joint extension over active extension and splinting of the MCP joints in flexion over splinting in extension. They conclude that no study to date evaluated the efficiency or suitability of any particular regime.

In 2001 Niels et al. from Copenhagen, Denmark undertook a retrospective study of 13 patients (41 joints) treated with dynamic splintage after replacing the metacarpophalangeal joint. Following the further analysis of a group of 9 patients (29 joints) treated without dynamic splintage they concluded that postoperative dynamic splintage seems to be more useful after replacement of the metacarpophalangeal joint when compared to simple splintage.

An alternate view was expressed by Burr et al. [4] from the United Kingdom in 2002. They undertook a prospective study to determine the results obtained using a static splinting regime as an alternative to a dynamic extension splintage. The study involved 15 patients with rheumatoid arthritis who had undergone metacarpophalangeal joint arthroplasty. The authors used measures of active arc of motion, together with ulnar deviation as well as a measure of activities of daily living to assess the outcome. They concluded that the initial results reinforced the clinical impression that a static splintage regime can be used instead of a dynamic outrigger.

Finally, Ring et al. [16] from Boston, USA investigated the use of continuous passing motion following MCP joint arthroplasty. A prospective trial was undertaken randomising patients to receive either continuous passive motion or a standard dynamic splint protocol. 25 patients in all were included in the study. Following measurements including range of motion, ulnar deviation, grip and lateral pinch strength to evaluate the outcome, they concluded that the incorporation of a continuous passive motion machine into postoperative rehabilitation did not offer a significant advantage.

3. Results

As discussed previously there are many methods for assessing the success of an arthroplasty. These include the effectiveness in delivering pain relief, movement, strength, improved function, cosmesis and of course survivalship. The latter is how long the arthroplasty will survive giving good results. In this section I will present the published data available for the various silastic implants, particularly the Swanson, focusing particularly on these markers of success.

Swanson [22] in an article in 1968, described the use of the flexible implant arthroplasty in the rheumatoid metacarpophalangeal joint. In that article he gave a description of the operative technique and postoperative rehabilitation programme. These techniques have formed the basis of metacarpophalangeal joint arthroplasty in this group of patients. In 1984 they republished results initially presented in 1982. They identified implant fractures in 12 out of 511 implants (2.35%) and a recurrent deformity in 65 (13%). They also obtained a range of motion averaging from 3° lack of extension to 65° of flexion at 29 months after surgery. Finally, the author reported an average improvement in grip and pinch strength. In a further article in 1986, they reported the long term bone response to silicone implants. By measuring cortical bone thickness they reported thickening of the bone around the implant stems in both the metacarpal and phalangeal metaphysis. As a result of this they concluded that the shape of the cortical bone in implant resection arthroplasty can be maintained and the bone thickness increased. Finally, in 1997 Swanson et al. [21] reported the successful use of press fit titanium circumferential grommets. These grommets were introduced to protect the flexible hinge implant mid section from sharp bony edges and shearing forces. They assessed the effectiveness by comparing the results of two groups of patients, one with and one without grommets. They identified 4 implant fractures (12.9%) in the non-grommet group and 1 (0.7%) in the grommet group.

Of particular note and more relevance however is the fact that there are numerous publications on this implant with short and long term follow up. These are from all four corners of the globe. For the short term the report by Blair et al. [2,3], reported a prospective analysis of 28 patients (115 implants) followed up for an average 4 1/2 years. The postoperative active motion of the joint averaged 43° from 30° of extension to 56° of flexion. This was an increase of 17° active movement from preoperative values. Unfortunately the ulnar drift recurred in 49 fingers (43%) and fracture of this spacer occurred in 24 joints (21%). Preoperative and postoperative key pinch and grip strength were unchanged while patient satisfaction was high. 71% of patients experienced significant pain relief and 68% felt they had better hand function. Finally 82% thought that the cosmetic appearance had improved.

In a similar study from Finland in 1986 Vahvanen and Viljakka [23] reported their results in 107 implants followed up for almost 45 months. Active movement reached 34°, ranging from 7° of extension to 41° of flexion. Although ulna deviation recurred in 31% of fingers fracture of the spacer was only seen in 4 joints. Again patient satisfaction was high, in that 27 out of 32 patients experienced significant pain relief, 31 hands (84%) felt that function had improved and all patients thought that the cosmetic appearance was better. Finally they did note however that on X-ray bone resorption around the stem was seen in 24%.

In 1986, Bieber et al. [1] from Baltimore, USA reported the results of 210 joints in 55 hands of patients with rheumatoid arthritis who had undergone Swanson MCP joint arthroplasty. Patients were followed up for between 2 and 8 years with an average of 5 1/4. In the initial postoperative period, the majority of patients expressed a strong subjective impression of improvement. Ulna drift improved from the preoperative average of 25° to less than 5°. Preoperative average extension deficit decreased from 56° to 10°, while the average range of motion increased from 17° to 51°. In the long term postoperative evaluation, the average ulna drift had increased to 12°, the average extension deficit had increased to 22° and the average range of motion had decreased to 39°. Grip strength and prehension did not significantly improve at either evaluation. In light of this the authors were able to conclude that while this procedure is useful for the correction of deformity, increasing range of movement of the fingers and the patients sense of well being, there was undoubtedly deterioration with time.

In 1997 Rothwell et al. [17] from New Zealand reported their results specifically using the Baltimore quantitative upper extremity function test in 21 consecutive rheumatoid patients who underwent metacarpophalangeal phalangeal joint arthroplasty. They demonstrated a progressive improvement in function, up to 3 to 4 years after surgery. They felt this was mainly attributable to an improvement in the ability to perform functions requiring pinch span and grip. This they felt was due largely to the correction of ulnar drift and change in metacarpophalangeal joint arc of motion.

Hansraj et al. [12] from New York again in 1997 reported their results of 348 implants in patients with rheumatoid arthritis. A smaller number of 170 were available for review at an average of 5.2-year follow up. Pain was found to be severe in 4% of the joints and with a further 3% having moderate discomfort. Indeed 39% had some slight discomfort, pain being completely absent in 54%. Movement preoperatively showed a flexion arc of 38° compared to 27° postoperatively. Functionally all patients reported they were able to feed themselves with the vast majority able to button clothes and write. Revision occurred in 11 cases for fracture. X-rays revealed that in 84% of patients there was some sclerosis of bone and 8% showing some resorption. Survivalship analysis revealed a 94% survivalship at 5 years, 93% at 7 years and 90% at 10 years using the end point of revision surgery.

To conclude and in the short term that is within 5 years of surgery, most studies report significant benefit from the silastic metacarpophalangeal joint arthroplasty. Complete pain relief is often seen in 70% to 80% of patients. Movement while usually better than preoperatively may not be significantly improved; generally the active range is from approximately 10° to 50°. Pinch and grip strength do not seem to be significantly effected, although most patients report an improvement in function. This can vary dependent upon the test used by somewhere in the region of 70% to 90%. With regard to ulnar deviation this undoubtedly recurs to a degree after surgery which may be due to several factors. Some studies report 25% to 30% recurrence rate within 5 years. Otherwise the vast majority of studies report a satisfaction rate of 80% plus, with a similar improvement in cosmesis. Finally the implant fracture rate again within this short time frame lies somewhere in the region of 5% to 20%.

For the medium to long term, again results have been reported from several corners of the globe. In 1983 Poulenas et al. [15] from Switzerland reported the results of 88 implants in 20 patients, followed up for between 7 and 15 years with an average follow up of 9. They reported a significant improvement in subjective hand movement and function in the majority of patients. Objectively no patient was experiencing discomfort with the average movement being 32°, which was equal for all fingers. This ranged between 13° and 47° of flexion. Residual ulnar deviation was 11°. With regard to complications these fell into two categories. Firstly, fracture of the prosthesis occurred in 23 cases, although none of these occurred with the newer HP prosthesis. Secondly, X-rays revealed that six of the prosthesis were dislocated. Overall they felt these results were very positive.

In 1993 Wilson et al. [24] from Chepstow in the United Kingdom reported their results in 77 patients who had undergone a total of 375 Swanson design silicone rubber implants. Using a combination of both clinical and postal evaluation ranging from 5 to 14 years after surgery, they noted that the vast majority of patients were satisfied with the outcome, more specifically the abolition of pain, correction of deformity and improved range of motion. They did note, however, that with time there was some increase in extension lag and some loss of active flexion. This ranged for the extension lag from 9° to 21° and for the flexion loss from 46° to 29°. Interestingly enough however, this reduction in the range of motion did not correlate with any functional deterioration. They also identified significant recurrent ulnar drift of more than 20° in 43% of patients. Radiologically 6 patients (17%) had subluxation/dislocation or fracture of the prosthesis. Generally however, the overall complication rate was low being less than 5%, with only 3% of prosthesis requiring revision or removal.

Schmidt et al. [18] from Germany in 1996 reported their results in 102 implants with an average 10.1-year follow up. They again confirmed a marked relief of pain in all patients with 75% reporting significant functional improvement. Again however range of motion decreased on average from 42° preoperatively to 36° postoperatively. Ulnar drift was corrected from an average of 34° preoperatively to 12° postoperatively. The average extensor deficit had an improvement of 33° at surgery to 11° at the time of follow up. Grip strength remained unchanged. Radiological findings included osteolysis surrounding 89.4% of the implants with 27.5% being broken. In a further study reported in 1997 they demonstrated some slight deterioration with time, specifically with ulnar deviation and function. Osteolysis described previously was also noted to be more prevalent. They also felt the additional use of titanium grommets reduced this reactive osteolysis and protected the implant.

Gellman et al. [8] from California, USA in 1997 reported a larger series of 264 patients who had undergone 901 Swanson silastic arthroplasties of the metacarpophalangeal joint. The average follow up was 8 years. Again they showed significant improvement in the correction of ulnar deviation from 45° preoperatively to 15° postoperatively. Active flexion averaged 40° preoperatively and 50° postoperatively, an increase of 10°. This involved an improvement in the extensor lag to 10° from 50°. The arc of movement ranged from 10° to 60° of flexion. Complications included delayed skin healing in 2%, superficial infection in 0.5% and deep infection in 3%. They also found prosthetic fracture in 14%. Subjectively most patients thought that their function had improved and that this was particularly attributable to the correction in ulnar deviation and improvement in extensor lag.

In 1999 Schmidt et al. [19,20] again reported updated results. This time in 28 patients (102 implants) with a mean follow up of 10 years. Again all patients reported pronounced subjective relief of pain and in 75% improved function. Movement more specifically active range of flexion decreased from 40° preoperatively to 35° postoperatively. Effectively this was due to an improvement in extension deficit. Again ulnar deviation was also improved, although grip strength was unchanged. Radiological examination revealed osteolysis around 89% of implants with 28% being broken. They concluded that material fatigue and sharp bony edges resulted in this osteolysis as well as implant fracture.

Chung et al. [5] in 2000 undertook a met-analysis of all published series from 1966 to 1999. While they were able to identify differences in the outcome, generally most research did demonstrate a correction of ulnar drift and an improvement in the arc of motion. They also found an improvement in pain and function, specifically activities of daily living with a high rate of patient satisfaction.

In 2003 Goldfarb and Stern [9] again from the USA reported their results of 208 arthroplasties in 52 hands (36 patients) operated on by one surgeon. The average follow up being 14 years. Results showed an improvement in the active arc of motion from 30° preoperatively to 46° after surgery, decreasing to 36° at long term follow up. The mean extension deficit for the metacarpophalangeal joint improved from 57° preoperatively to 11° immediately after surgery, worsening to 23° at final follow up. Similarly, ulnar drift improved from 26° preoperatively to less than 5° postoperatively, averaging 16° at long term follow up. Implant fractures were associated with increased ulnar drift. Bone reaction adjacent to the implant was demonstrated by bone shortening in most patients and erosions in 29%. 130 implants (63%) were broken and 45 (22%) more were deformed at the time of final follow up. Patient satisfaction and function rated 38% and only 27% of hands were pain free. Ulnar drift was associated with decreased patient satisfaction particularly with regard to cosmetic appearance.

In 2003 results from Wrightington Hospital in 381 patients with rheumatoid arthritis reported a total of 1336 implants over a 17-year period. Implant failure was defined as either revision or fracture of the implant as seen on X-ray. Using both these criteria as an end point the survivalship at 17 years using Kaplan–Meier was 63% (Fig. 5). On radiographs 2/3 of the implant were seen to be broken. Factors which improve survival include soft tissue rebalancing, cross intrinsic transfer and realignment at the time of surgery. Surgery to the thumb and proximal interphalangeal joint had a deleterious effect and the use of grommets did not seem to protect the implant from fracture. Finally the alignment of the radiocarpal joint seemed pivotal.

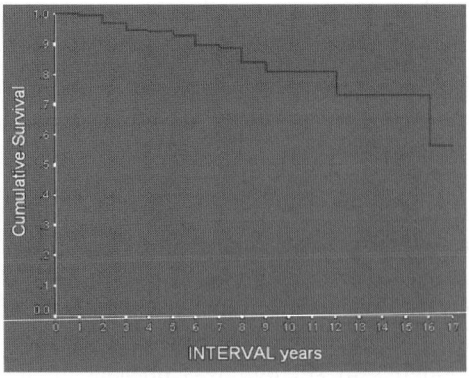

Fig. 5. Kaplan–Meier survivalship.

By way of summary for the longer term, that is 10 years or more, several large series indicate that patient satisfaction remains high with this prosthesis and generally there is a low complication and revision rate. It is however generally accepted that movement, both flexion and extension, diminishes with time; ulna deviation can also progress. Surprisingly this does not seem to result in a marked diminution in function. Radiologically an increasing number of the implants fracture with time and undoubtedly this is associated with a recurrence of ulna deviation. Again however, the majority of patients do not require revision.

4. Complications

The principal complications of metacarpophalangeal joint replacements are similar to all other arthroplasties. However, silicone itself can lead to particular problems. In 1975 Ferlic et al. [7] from Denver, Colorado reported a series of complications in 162 metacarpophalangeal silicone prosthesis inserted between 1967 and 1973. Of this group 15 had fractured, 2 were associated with infection and there was one case of skin necrosis. Recurrence of ulnar drift occurred in 4 hands. Overall 3 prosthesis had to be removed.

In 1981 Groff et al. [11] reported the case of a patient with rheumatoid arthritis who had had a previous silicone MCP joint replacement, who developed an axillary lymphade-nopathy secondary to silicone particles. Finally, Jozsa et al. [13] from Budapest, Hungary in 1993 reported the histological examination of material removed from around a silicone implant at revision surgery. They were able to identify both in the synovial tissue and in the intramedullary bone cavity the presence of foreign body granulation tissue. This inflammatory tissue was characterised by mono-nuclear cells and in addition in one patient mild eosinophilia. All specimens contained a particulate foreign body material which was felt to be silicone, particles ranging from 4 to 300 μm in size. They concluded that while the clinical incidence was low, there was significant potential for further problems with this type of implant.

In the authors personal opinion after undertaking a significant number of silicone metacarpophalangeal arthroplasties over the years, the development of silicone synovitis at this site is quite rare. In over 1500 joint replacements undertaken at Wrightington only four implants have been revised for this complication (Fig. 6).

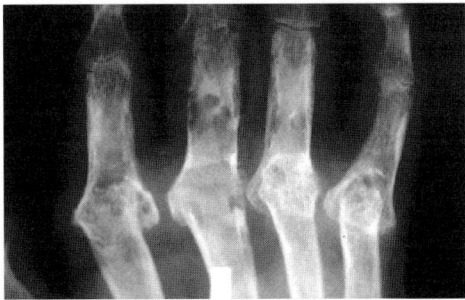

Fig. 6. Silicone synovitis.

Infection has also been reported although again its incidence is low. In 1992 Golz et al. [10] from Los Angeles, California reported a case of late infection around a metacarpophalangeal joint silicone implant in a patient 10 years after insertion. The infection was treated by removal of the implant and a thorough irrigation and debridement of the wound. The infecting organism being *Staphylococcus aureus*. Finally Dunkley and Leslie [6] in 1997 reported a case of candida infection in a silicone metacarpophalangeal joint replacement. Again in the author's experience infection of these silicone implants is again quite rare and can be easily treated by removal with debridement/curettage as appropriate. The patient should of course also be treated by a long course of initially intravenous and subsequent oral antibiotics. The results of such an excision arthroplasty are often quite gratifying.

Another more worrying complication is skin necrosis immediately after surgery. As can be appreciated as most of the patients undergoing this procedure have some form of inflammatory arthritis, the skin can be very thin and as a consequence easily damaged. In addition if the patients are taking steroids this can lead to a delay in healing. If poor surgical technique is added to this then of course there is a risk of skin necrosis. In the author's experience this has occurred predominantly with a transverse incision. Treatment of this is very much dependent on the extent of the necrosis. Generally however, the patient returns to the operating room and the dead skin excised. If this is a small area and implants are not exposed the wound can be allowed to heal by primary intention. If however the defect is larger and an implant can be seen, then either a skin graft or flap cover is required.

Another complication that can be seen in the early postoperative period is dislocation. By this it is meant that one of the stems of the silastic implant can dislocate out of the shafts of either the metacarpal or phalanx. This is often manifested clinically by a swelling in the palm, the diagnosis being confirmed by a radiographic examination. Treatment of this again would take the form of revision surgery with reinsertion of the stem. Care should be taken however, as a cause of this dislocation can be inadequate soft tissue release or bony resection leading to mal-alignment of the metacarpal and phalange. This should be addressed at the time of revision surgery. For the two-part implant instability is a more common problem. This can occur for a variety of reasons, particularly poor surgical decision making and technique. Patently if there is significant bone loss at the metacarpophalangeal joint and preoperative instability, it is likely that the same problem will remain after the procedure. It would seem sensible in this particular clinical scenario to choose a hinged or linked implant. At surgery insertion of a two-piece implant requires a different surgical philosophy from that of a silastic implant. The latter is effectively an excision arthroplasty, with quite radical removal of bone and release of soft tissues were appropriate, whereas the former is more like a conventional arthroplasty with limited bone resection and preservation of restraining structures. Obviously if the surgeon is overzealous in his approach this can precipitate instability. Experience with regard to management of an unstable two-piece implant is however limited and certainly there is little published. Effectively there are two surgical options. The first is some sort of soft tissue reconstruction and the second revision to a hinged or linked implant. The author has had limited success with the former but some success with revision to a silastic linked implant.

A somewhat later problem is stiffness of the metacarpophalangeal joint. It should be noted that this can be seen with both silastic and two-part replacements. While this is not a catastrophe in so much that a pain free, stable, well aligned joint can be of significant value to the patient, particularly in the presence of a functioning proximal interphalangeal joint, the results can be disappointing to both patients and surgeons alike. Reasons for this stiffness often include poor surgical release at the time of surgery, adhesions around the flexor or extensor tendons, poor patient cooperation with therapy and finally good function of the proximal interphalangeal joint. More specifically it does appear that in patients who have good if not full flexion of the proximal interphalangeal joints rarely require full flexion of the metacarpophalangeal joints. This fact can be incorporated into therapy programmes in so much that blocking the proximal interphalangeal joint movement during therapy can enhance metacarpophalangeal joint movement. If the patient is dissatisfied with the movement of their metacarpophalangeal joint, I believe the only option is again revision surgery. However in the author's experience while this surgery has been attempted followed by a course of intensive hand therapy, results are often disappointing.

The next potential complication is recurrent ulnar drift (Fig. 7). In the author's experience and from a review of literature it does appear that in patients with inflammatory arthritis recurrent ulnar drift is inevitable. Obviously however, if this recurs significantly in the first few months after surgery, this will result in a poor cosmetic appearance. There are many factors leading to ulnar drift, the paramount among them being radial deviation of the radiocarpal joint. If the patient has radial deviation of the wrist prior to surgery, in the author's opinion this should be addressed if possible. If the patient develops this deformity after MCP joint surgery then again any wrist deformity will have to be corrected prior to any revision surgery. As stated previously in the Results there are a number of other factors leading to the development of this deformity, including surgery to the thumb and arthrodesis of the proximal interphalangeal joint. Plainly however, these operations are undertaken for different reasons and sometimes cannot be avoided. Again if revision surgery is undertaken it is important that adequate soft tissue release and rebalancing is

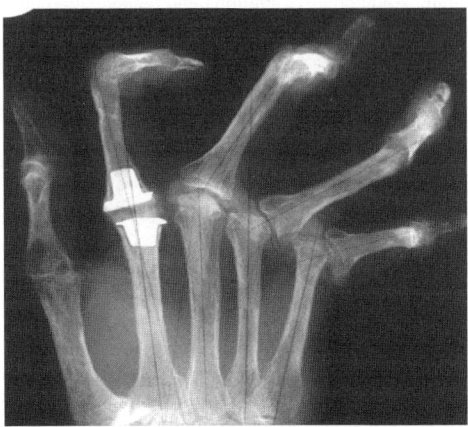

Fig. 7. Recurrent ulna drift.

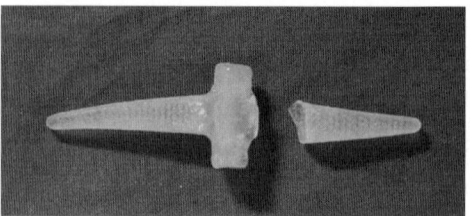

Fig. 8. Fractured silicone implant.

undertaken. In the author's institution this would include a cross intrinsic transfer or at the very least reconstruction of the radial collateral ligament.

Finally, silicone implants can fracture (Fig. 8) and indeed again as has already been stated in the Results fracture of the implant is almost inevitable. In a series from Wrightington Hospital with a long term follow up at 16 years almost two thirds of the implants were felt to be fractured on X-ray. Interestingly enough the majority of these patients did not require revision, in that they did not seem to experience increasing pain, movement was retained although many did develop increased ulnar deviation. If surgery is required however, then as with the recurrent ulnar deviation further bony resection is undertaken together with soft tissue release/rebalancing as appropriate. Obviously a new implant is inserted.

References

[1] E.J. Bieber, A.J. Weiland, S. Volenec-Dowling, Silicone-rubber implant arthroplasty of the metacarpophalangeal joints for rheumatoid arthritis, J Bone Joint Surg Vol. 68-A (No. 2) (1986 (Feb)) 206–209.
[2] W.F. Blair, D.G. Shurr, J.A. Buckwalter, Metacarpophalangeal joint arthroplasty with a metallic hinged prosthesis, Metacarpophalangeal Joint Arthro 184 (1984) 156–163.
[3] W.F. Blair, D.G. Shurr, J.A. Buckwalter, Metacarpophalangeal joint implant arthroplasty with a silastic spacer, J Bone and Joint Surg 66A (No. 3) (1984) 365–370.
[4] N. Burr, A.L. Pratt, P.J. Smith, An alternative splinting and rehabilitation protocol for metacarpophalangeal joint arthroplasty in patients with rheumatoid arthritis, J Hand Ther 15 (2002) 41–47.
[5] K.C. Chung, et al., Patient outcomes following swanson silastic metacarpophalangeal joint arthroplasty in the rheumatoid hand: a systematic overview, J. Rheumatol. 27 (2000) 1395–1402.
[6] A.B. Dunkley, I.J. Leslie, Candida infection of a silicone metacarpophalangeal arthroplasty, J Hand Surg 22B (3) (1997) 423–424.
[7] D.C. Ferlic, M.L. Clayton, M. Holloway, Complications of silicone implant surgery in the metacarpophalangeal joint, J Bone Joint Surg 57-A (1975) 991–994.
[8] H. Gellman, et al., Silastic metacarpophalangeal joint arthroplasty in patients with rheumatoid arthritis, Clinical Ortho and Related Research No. 342 (1997) 16–21.
[9] C.A. Goldfarb, P.J. Stern, Metacarpophalangeal joint arthroplasty in rheumatoid arthritis, J Bone and Joint Surg 85 (10) (2003) 1869–1878.
[10] R. Golz, S.H. Kuschner, H. Gellman, Sequential infection of silicone metacarpophalangeal joint arthroplasties resulting from skin breakdown, J Hand Surg 17A (1992) 150–152.
[11] G.D. Groff, A.R. Schned, T.H. Taylor, Silicone-induced adenopathy eight years after metacarpophalangeal arthroplasty, Arthritis and Rheumatism Vol. 24 (1981) 1578–1581.
[12] K.K. Hansraj, et al., Swanson metacarpophalangeal joint arthroplasty in patients with rheumatoid arthritis, Clinical Ortho and Related Research No. 342 (1997) 11–15.

[13] L. Józsa, A. Renner, Frenyó., Silicone-induced synovial and osseal granuloma following metacarpopha-langeal and carpal arthroplasty, Zentralbl. Pathol 139 (1993) 313–319.

[14] Massy-Westropp, J. Krishnan, Postoperative therapy after metacarpophalangeal arthroplasty, J Hand Ther 16 (2003) 311–314.

[15] I. Poulenas, C. Simonetta, D.V. Egloff, Long-term results from metacarpophalangeal arthroplasty, Ann. Chir. Main 2 (2) (1983) 160–167.

[16] D. Ring, B.P. Simmons, M. Hayes, Continuous passive motion following metacarpophalangeal joint arthroplasty, J Hand Surg 23A (1998) 505–511.

[17] A.G. Rothwell, K.J. Cragg, L.B. O'Neill, Hand function following silastic arthroplasty of the metacarpophalangeal joints in the rheumatoid hand, J Hand Surg 22B (1) (1997) 90–93.

[18] V.K. Schmidt, R.K. Miehlke, K. Witt, Long-term follow up of mp-joint arthroplasty with swanson silastic spacers. Handchir, Mikrochir. Plast. Chir 28 (1996) 254–264.

[19] K. Schmidt, et al., Ten-year follow-up of silicone arthroplasty of the metacarpophalangeal joints in rheumatoid hands, Scand J Plast ReconstrHand Surg 33 (1999) 433–438.

[20] K. Schmidt, et al., The effect of the additional use of grommets in silicone implant arthroplasty of the metacarpophalangeal joints, J Hand Surg 24B (5) (1999) 561–564.

[21] A.B. Swanson, G. de Groot Swanson, H. Ishikawa, Use of grommets for flexible implant resection arthroplasty of the metacarpophalangeal joint, Clin Ortho and related research No. 342 (1997) 22–33.

[22] A.B. Swanson, Silicone rubber implants for replacement of arthritic or destroyed joints in the hand, Surgical Clinics of North America Vol. 48 (No. 5) (1968 (Oct)) 1113–1127.

[24] V. Vahvanen, T. Viljakka, Silicone rubber implant arthroplasty of the metacarpophalangeal joint in rheumatoid arthritis: a follow-up study of 32 patients, J Hand Surg 11A (1986) 333–339.

[25] Y.G. Wilson, P.J. Sykes, N.S. Niranjan, Long-term follow up of swanson's silastic arthroplasty of the metacarpophalangeal joints in rheumatoid arthritis, J Hand Surg 18B (1993) 81–91.

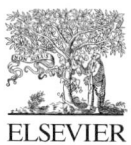

International Congress Series 1295 (2006) 144–153

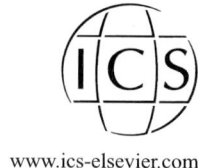

www.ics-elsevier.com

How I do it—MP joint arthroplasty

Christer Sollerman

Sahlgrenska Universitetssjukhuset, Handkir, kliniken, S-413 45, Gotenberg, Sweden

Keywords: Human hand; Reconstructive hand surgery; MCP-joint arthroplasty; Rheumatoid arthritis

1. Introduction

The human hand is used as a prehensile organ, the function of which is very important for both activities of daily living and working capacity. Restoring hand function after injuries or disabling diseases is therefore a major task in reconstructive hand surgery. Hand function is based upon certain properties of the hand, which can be characterized as: freedom from pain, functional sensibility, stability and range of motion of joints with proper grip strength. These properties are listed in order of significance, freedom from pain and tactile sensibility being more important than range of motion and strength. This fact forms the basis for many of the surgical procedures used in rheumatoid arthritis, e.g. when arthrodesis of a joint improves hand function through transforming a painful unstable joint into a pain-free and stable fusion. The loss of joint motion after such a procedure is for certain joints, i.e. the metacarpo-phalangeal joint of the thumb, of minor importance compared to the improvement due to stability and pain relief. Other joints, however, such as the MCP-joints of the fingers, need range of motion to enable good grip function. When the MCP-joints of the fingers have been destroyed causing pain, deformity and stiffness, endoprosthetic replacement is the principal surgical option, in order to preserve as much range of motion as possible. The appearance and function of the hand, however, is also a part of the body language, affecting social life and interpersonal relations to a very significant degree. In our western region the hands are, together with the face, the only parts of the body that are not covered by clothes, which make deformities of the hand most obvious to the surrounding. Hand deformities in rheumatoid arthritis are therefore not only a prehensile handicap affecting occupational capacity and activities of daily living, but

E-mail address: christer.sollerman@orthop.gu.se.

might also lead to a psychosocial disability. The most common indication for MCP-joint arthroplasty in rheumatoid arthritis (RA) is ulnar deviation and volar subluxation of the fingers, ulnar drift (Fig. 1). Ulnar drift affects more than 50% of patients with RA and is regarded as the most characteristic deformity of rheumatic disease. Some patients with ulnar drift experience pain in their MCP-joints, which is the main indication for MCP-joint arthroplasty, others complain of loss of hand function. Functional complaints are often related to the flexion contracture of volar subluxated MCP-joints resulting in an impaired opening grip. Patients may experience difficulties in grasping large objects, shaking hands or washing the face. The main goal for surgical treatment of ulnar drift therefore could be defined as pain relief, improving MCP-joint extension and correction of the ulnar deviation. The timing and type of surgical procedure, as well as the expected result, should be discussed with the patient in detail. Rheumatoid patients are often well informed about different surgical options and must be allowed to have a major influence on the decision whether surgery should be performed, or not. Such a discussion is preferably performed in a team setting consisting of hand surgeon, rheumatologist, physical or occupational therapist. Surgical treatment in RA has a long tradition, but many of the commonly used procedures are based on clinical experience and uncontrolled data. In a meta-analysis by the Swedish Council on Technology Assessment in Health Care [19] the main conclusion was that better documentation of both new and established surgical procedures is needed. This is especially important in MCP-joint arthroplasty, when new procedures and new implants are introduced.

2. Surgical procedures

The surgical options intended to improve function of the MCP-joints of the fingers include tenosynovectomy, tendon transfer or tendon repair, soft tissue stabilizing procedures, arthro-synovectomy, arthrodesis and arthroplasty.

The indication for surgery is based mainly on symptoms and clinical findings rather than radiographic appearance. A classification of the clinical deformity into three stages was made by Fearnley [5] and is still useful when different treatment options are discussed. A staging of the radiographic destruction is also essential for the choice between various surgical alternatives. According to Larsen-Dale-Eek, rheumatoid joint destruction is commonly classified in stages I–VI; stage I corresponds to a normal radiographic appearance, stage VI corresponds to a totally destroyed joint [12]. Endoprosthetic replacement of the MCP-joints is indicated in Fearnley stage 3 (joint contracture) and with radiographic changes corresponding to Larsen stage III or worse. The recently introduced non-constrained implants for MCP-joint replacement are, however, most useful in earlier stages. Isolated synovectomy of the MCP-joints was a frequent procedure in the past, but is now usually performed as an adjunct to soft tissue stabilizing procedures. Fusion of the MCP-joint of the index finger is sometimes performed in conjunction with arthroplasty of the remaining fingers, in order to achieve improved stability in lateral pinch.

3. The MCP-joint and ulnar drift

The MCP-joints of the fingers are ball-in-socket joints allowing range of motion from $1°$ to $20°$ of hyperextension to $90°$ of flexion. In an extended position $25°$ of ulnar-radial deviation is possible, while the joints become laterally stable in the flexed position. The range of motion of the MCP-joints is important, both for opening the hand and for the grasping of objects. Lateral stability is needed, especially in the index finger when used in the lateral pinch.

Ulnar drift and volar subluxation are often both functionally and psychologically a dominating problem for the RA patient. In most cases ulnar drift causes impaired prehensile function with impaired extension capacity resulting in difficulties to open the hand. In some cases, the pinch grip between the thumb and the finger tips is lost, leaving the lateral pinch between the thumb and the radial side of the index finger as the only remaining grip for manipulation [26]. Even if the prehensile function of the hand is preserved, patients often experience ulnar drift as cosmetically disturbing, and strongly urge a surgical correction.

The development of ulnar drift is caused by:

– radial deviation of the wrist joint leading to hand scoliosis with secondary ulnar deviation of the fingers (Fig. 1);
– tenosynovitis of the flexor tendon sheath leading to weakening of annular ligaments with subsequent ulnarly directed forces of the flexor tendons onto the index and middle fingers;
– synovitis of MCP-joints leading to weakening of the transverse ligaments of the extensor tendon "hood" with subsequent ulnar luxation of the extensor tendons;
– common use of lateral pinch in which the thumb creates ulnarly directed forces to the radial side of the index finger.

These different forces produce ulnar deviation of the fingers and volar subluxation of the proximal phalanx from the metacarpal heads, which are a main part of the deformity and the cause of extension loss of the MCP-joints.

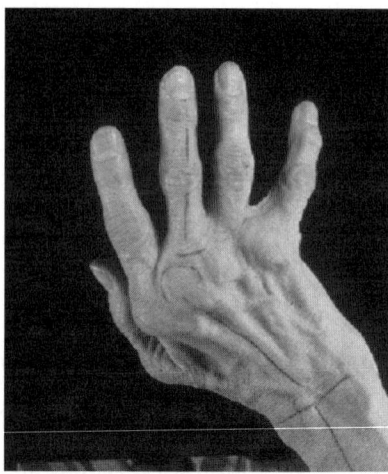

Fig. 1. Rheumatoid hand with ulnar drift.

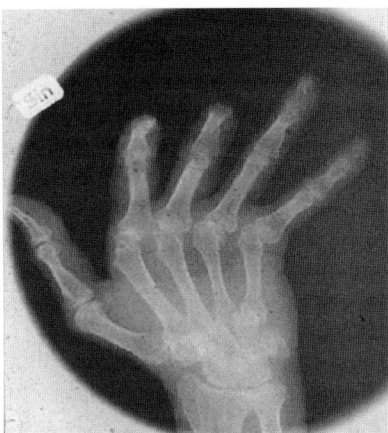

Fig. 2. Radiographic appearance of ulnar drift Fearnley stage 3.

Ulnar drift is classified into three stages according to Fearnley [5]. The early stage (Fearnley 1: active reduction is possible=minor deformity which might be corrected by the muscle activity of the hand itself) is often treated with dynamic splinting with rubber bands counteracting both the ulnar deviation and the volar subluxation of the fingers. In the next stage (Fearnley 2: passive reduction is possible=more severe deformity which can be corrected with splints or with the help of the contralateral hand) the MCP-joints are still radiographically normal and soft tissue surgical procedures might be used to correct the ulnar deviation. In the last stage (Fearnley 3: fixed deformity combined with subluxation and radiographic destruction of the MCP-joints), soft tissue procedures are no longer successful; arthroplasty of the MCP-joints is the recommended surgical correction (Fig. 2).

4. Arthroplasty of the MCP-joints

The first reported surgical procedure using an endoprosthesis for replacement of the MCP-joints was performed in the beginning of the 1950s and since then a variety of endoprostheses have been presented [3]. The joint mechanism might be constrained using a polymer, such as silicone, as the flexible hinge, or non-constrained using a ball-in-socket concept. The stem of the endoprosthesis might be fixed into the bone marrow channels, with or without cement, or it might be encapsulated by soft tissues as the main fixation. Non-cemented implant stems might, under certain conditions, be strongly anchored to the surrounding bone tissue, i.e. osseointegration. The term osseointegration has been frequently used when pure titanium is fixated to the bone tissue [4].

5. Silicone implants

Arthroplasty using silicone implants was introduced by Swanson and has for more than 30 years been the gold standard for endoprosthetic replacement of the MCP-joints [10,22]. The concept is based on a flexible silicone spacer with proximally and distally directed stems (Fig. 3), which after resection of the metacarpal head are introduced into the marrow channels of the metacarpal bone and the proximal phalanx, respectively. The spacer is

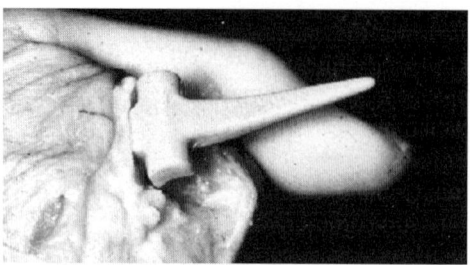

Fig. 3. Silicone implant of Swanson type.

subsequently "encapsulated" by a firm fibrous capsule, which serves as the main implant fixation [21]. The radial collateral ligaments, at least for the index finger, are reinserted to bone before implantation of the spacers. With the Swanson arthroplasty immediate pain relief, proper correction of deformity and adequate range of motion is often obtained. With time, however, bony reactions tend to occur around the implants, both as new bone formation, or as bone resorption, due to movements between implant and bone [7]. The range of motion might deteriorate due to subsidence of the implants into the surrounding bone. Silicone particle induced synovitis has mainly been described around silicone implants in larger joints, but it can occasionally occur in MCP-joints [18]. Range of motion varying between 25° and 66° has been reported, which usually is enough for a functional grip when the PIP-joint movement is preserved. More important than proper range of motion is the shift of the motion arc from a flexed to an extended position, which improves the opening grip [20,25]. High fracture rates of the silicone spacers are often considered as a disadvantage of the method, and long-term studies have shown up to 58% fractures 14 years after surgery [6]. Titanium bone liners, so called grommets, were introduced by Swanson to protect the implant from wearing against sharp bony edges (Figs. 4 and 5). The advantage of using grommets in routine arthroplasties has been debated [9], but they are useful in reinforcing the surrounding bone when pronounced bone resorption is present, for example in revision procedures.

A new design of silicone implants was introduced by Sutter (now Avanta) in which the implant surface against the resected bone ends is larger in order to prevent subsidence of the implant, and the axis of motion placed more volarly to improve the range of motion (Fig. 6). A fracture rate of 45% in patients followed for more than 3 years has been reported with this implant [1]. A prospective randomized comparison between Swanson

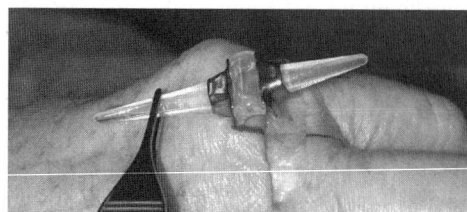

Fig. 4. Swanson silicone implant with titanium grommets prior to implantation.

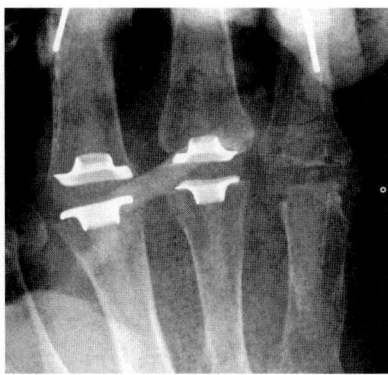

Fig. 5. Swanson silicone implants with titanium grommets in MCP III–IV, without grommets in MCP V.

and Avanta implants showed no significant difference between the implants, but a fracture rate of 13% and 20%, respectively, after 2 years [16].

In order to improve results and minimize the risk of implant fracture, pre-bent implants have been introduced to improve the biomechanical properties of the implants. Prospective studies will be necessary to show whether this design will improve long-term results or not.

Other polymeric materials such as polyurethane have been used in limited series as an alternative to silicone, but experience is limited [23].

Silicone arthroplasty of the MCP-joints is, in spite of the obvious disadvantages with silicone, a rewarding procedure as most patients are satisfied with the functional and cosmetic result. Most surgeons recommend this technique as the standard procedure for MCP-joint replacement in rheumatoid arthritis because of its reliable results.

6. Silicone implants with titanium screw fixation

Much of the problems of using silicone implants are created by the movement between implant and bone producing implant wear. A more stable fixation of the implant stems would avoid this problem. Stable fixation of implants might be obtained by using titanium fixators for anchoring the implant to bone. The osseointegration concept was introduced

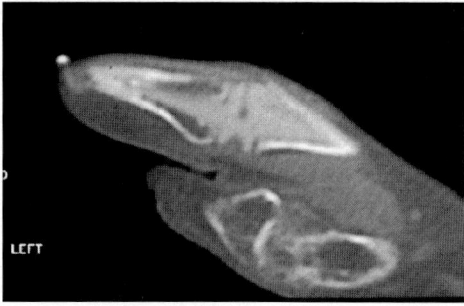

Fig. 6. CT-scan of Avanta silicone implant showing broad surfaces preventing implant subsidence.

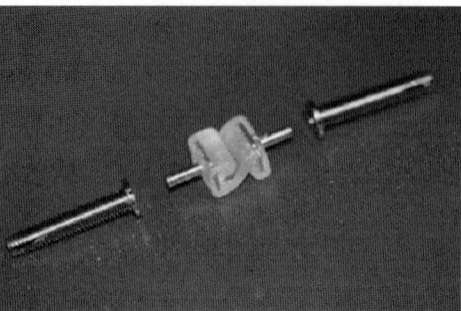

Fig. 7. Silicone implant with titanium fixtures ad modum Brånemark.

by Brånemark in the late 1960s, and has been used extensively for fixation of artificial teeth [4]. Results from osseointegrated MCP-implants were first reported by Hagert, but the joint mechanism in this series was complicated and the clinical results were less successful [8]. In another series a constrained hinge joint made of silicone with titanium stems anchored to titanium screw-shaped fixtures in the marrow channels of the surrounding bone was used (Fig. 7). Preliminary results showed 100% osseointegration (measured from X-ray examinations) and excellent clinical results [13]. The fracture rate of the silicone is, however, a problem with this implant design, 6% silicone fractures reported after 2.5 years, but the rate did tend to increase further with time [15]. The use of alternate materials for the hinge mechanism might improve long-term results. Prototypes using polyurethane or a metal spring for the hinge are now being tested (G. Lundborg, personal communication) (Fig. 8).

7. Non-constrained implants

The gold standard in replacement of the hip and the knee is arthroplasty with non-constrained implants, and numerous studies have shown this concept being most successful in large joint replacements. This concept has also been tried in MCP-joint arthroplasty, but with less success. A non-constrained implant with a metal ball articulating in a plastic socket with implant stems fixed to surrounding bone with the help of bone cement was first described by Steffee [24]. Extensive periarticular ectopic bone formation and loosening of the distal stem have contributed to a very limited use of this implant. Other similar designs have failed to correct deformity, and recurrence of ulnar drift was common after such procedures.

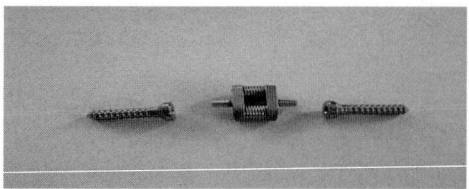

Fig. 8. Hinge mechanism with parallel metal springs for MCP-joint replacement (Biospring®). Published with permission from G. Lundborg.

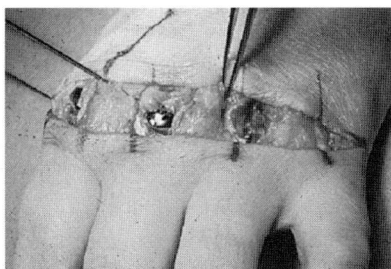

Fig. 9. Surgical view of exposed MCP-joints with SR-implants.

In 1983, Beckenbaugh presented a non-constrained implant for the MCP-joint made from a new material called pyrolytic carbon [2]. This material has biomechanical properties similar to bone and might be fixated to the surrounding bone without cement in a procedure similar to osseointegration. The implant has a ball-in-socket design with very shallow surfaces with both components made of pyrocarbon. Good results have been reported in osteoarthritis patients [17], but studies in rheumatoid arthritis are not yet available.

A non-constrained implant, with a metal ball articulating against polyethylene, has recently been introduced by the Avanta Company in cooperation with the Mayo Clinic [11]. The metal component has flails intended to improve implant stability and this implant should be used with cement (Fig. 9).

Early reports and personal experience with non-constrained implants reveal good results in terms of range of motion, pain relief and correction of ulnar drift (Fig. 10), in most cases better than with silicone implants. Recurrence of ulnar drift has, however, been reported with all kinds of non-constrained implants, as the soft tissues in most patients with rheumatoid arthritis are not stable enough to preserve lateral stability. Non-constrained implants should probably not be used in advanced deformities, but might be considered in single joint replacement or in an early stage of ulnar drift. Long-term studies are needed before non-constrained implants can be recommended as a standard procedure.

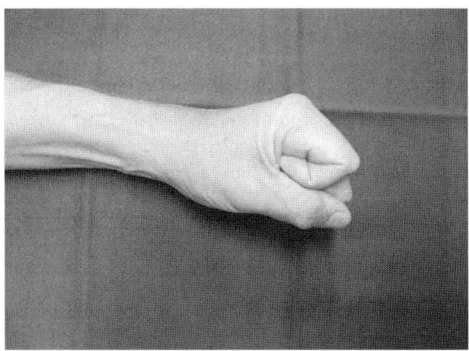

Fig. 10. MCP-joint flexion 6 months after arthroplasty with SR-implants.

8. Post-operative rehabilitation

Post-operative therapy has been considered crucial for gaining good results after MCP-joint arthroplasty. Swanson recommended the use of early mobilization with dynamic splints during the post-operative period [21]. A specialized team with physical and occupational therapists is often needed in the post-operative period to design proper splints and supervise the therapy.

Splints are custom-made from various plastic materials by occupational therapists. Static splints are used for immobilization. Dynamic splints use rubber bands acting on the fingers in order to counteract muscle forces, correct deformities and to facilitate range of motion. After silicone arthroplasty, a dynamic splint with rubber bands providing radial traction of the fingers is used for 6–8 weeks post-operatively. Such a splint should allow flexion–extension exercises to be performed 10–15 times a day. A static splint is used at night, often for prolonged periods of several months post-operatively.

Non-constrained implants with less inherent stability than constrained implants need immobilization after MCP-joint arthroplasty for 1–2 weeks before exercises with dynamic splints are initiated.

As the incidence of silicone fractures has become more widely known, many surgeons prefer more protective post-operative protocols with immobilization of the MCP-joints during 2–3 weeks before motion is allowed. Some surgeons prefer using intermittent immobilization combined with passive exercises during the entire post-operative period. Whether such a regime will result in improved implant survival or impaired range of motion is still to be evaluated [14].

References

[1] R.L. Bass, P.J. Stern, J.G. Nairus, High implant fracture incidence with Sutter silicone metacarpophalangeal joint arthroplasty, J. Hand Surg. 21A (5) (1996) 813–818.
[2] R.D. Beckenbaugh, Preliminary experience with a noncemented nonconstrained total joint arthroplasty for the metacarpophalangeal joint, Orthopedics 6 (8) (1983) 962–965.
[3] D.J. Beevers, B.B. Seedhom, Metacarpophalangeal joint prostheses, J. Hand Surg. 20B (1995) 125–136.
[4] P.I. Brånemark, et al., Intraosseus anchorage of dental prosthesis: I. Experimental studies, Scand. J. Plast. Reconstr. Surg. 3 (1969) 81–100.
[5] G.R. Fearnley, Ulnar deviation of fingers, Ann. Rheum. Dis. 10 (1951) 126–136.
[6] C.A. Goldfarb, P.J. Stern, Metacarpophalangeal joint arthroplasty in rheumatoid arthritis, A long-term assessment, J. Bone Jt. Surg. 85A (10) (2003) 1869–1878.
[7] C.-G. Hagert, et al., Metacarpophalangeal joint implants: I. Roentgenographic study of the silastic finger joint implant, Swanson design, Scand. J. Plast. Reconstr. Surg. 9 (1975) 147–157.
[8] C.-G. Hagert, et al., Metacarpophalangeal joint replacement with osseointegrated endoprostheses, Scand. J. Plast. Reconstr. Hand Surg. 20 (1986) 207–218.
[9] M. Horlbeck, H. Thabe, Initial results following implantation of silastic wrist joint prostheses in patients with chronic polyarthritis with additional use of titanium grommets, Handchir. Mikrochir. Plast. Chir. 21 (1) (Jan 1989) 48–50.
[10] D. Kirschenbaum, et al., Arthroplasty of the metacarpophalangeal joints with use of silicone rubber implants in patients who have rheumatoid arthritis, J. Bone Jt. Surg. 75A (1993) 3–12.
[11] P.L. Kung, et al., Intrinsic stability of an unconstrained metacarpophalangeal joint implant, Clin. Biomech. 18 (2) (2003) 119–125.

[12] A. Larsen, K. Dale, M. Eek, Radiographic evaluation of rheumatoid arthritis and related conditions by standard reference films, Acta Radiol., Diagn. 18 (1977) 481–491.

[13] G. Lundborg, P.-I. Brånemark, I. Carlsson, Metacarpophalangeal joint arthroplasty based on the osseointegration concept, J. Hand Surg. 18 B (1993) 693–703.

[14] N. Massy-Westropp, J. Krishnan, Postoperative therapy after metacarpophalangeal arthroplasty, J. Hand Ther. 16 (4) (2003) 311–314.

[15] K. Möller, et al., Osseointegrated silicone implants, 18 patients with 57 MCP joints followed for 2 years, Acta Orthop. Scand. 70 (2) (1999) 109–115.

[16] K. Möller, et al., Avanta versus Swanson silicone implants in the MCP-joints—a prospective, randomized comparison of 30 patients followed for 2 years, J. Hand Surg. 30B (1) (2005) 8–13.

[17] V.A. Nunez, N.D. Citron, Short-term results of the Ascension pyrolytic carbon metacarpophalangeal joint replacement arthroplasty for osteoarthritis, Chir. Main 24 (3–4) (2005) 161–164.

[18] C. Peimer, et al., Reactive synovitis after silicone arthroplasty, J. Hand Surg. 11A (5) (1986) 624–638.

[19] SBU-TSCoTAiHC, Rheumatic diseases—surgical treatment, Scand. J. Rheumatol. 28 (Suppl. 110) (1999).

[20] J.K. Stanley, A.R. Tolat, Long-term results of Swanson silastic arthroplasty in the rheumatoid wrist, J. Hand Surg. 18B (1993) 381–388.

[21] A.B. Swanson, Finger joint replacement by silicone rubber implants and the concept of implant fixation by encapsulation, Ann. Rheum. Dis. 28 (5) (1969) 47–55 (Suppl.).

[22] A.B. Swanson, Flexible implant arthroplasty for arthritic finger joints: rationale, technique and results of treatment, J. Bone Jt. Surg. 54A (3) (1972) 435–455.

[23] C.J. Sollerman, M. Geijer, Polyurethane versus silicone for endoprosthetic replacement of the metacarpophalangeal joints in rheumatoid arthritis, Scand. J. Plast. Reconstr. Hand Surg. 30 (1996) 145–150.

[24] A. Steffee, R. Beckenbaugh, R. Lindsheid, The development, technique and early results of total joint replacement for the metacarpophalangeal joint of the fingers, Orthopedics 4 (1981) 175–180.

[25] Y.G. Wilson, P.J. Sykes, N.S. Niranjan, Long-term follow-up of Swanson's silastic arthoplasty of the metacarpophalngeal joints in rheumatoid arthritis, J. Hand Surg. 18B (1) (1993) 81–91.

[26] R.L. Wilson, E.R. Carlblom, The rheumatoid metacarpophalangeal joint, Hand Clin. 5 (2) (1989) 223–237.

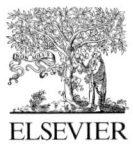

International Congress Series 1295 (2006) 154–157

ELSEVIER

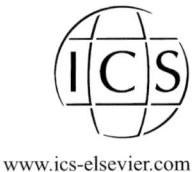

www.ics-elsevier.com

Assessment and management of swan neck deformity

S.L. Knight

St James's University Hospital, Beckett Street, LEEDS LS9 7TF, UK

Abstract. Development of the swan neck deformity in rheumatoid arthritis is a complicated process caused by abnormalities in the structure of the PIP joint and abnormalities in the forces on the joints of the finger. Surgical treatment relies on controlling or reversing these abnormalities. Four clinical groups are described and the indications for surgical treatment of each group are presented. © 2006 Published by Elsevier B.V.

Keywords: Swan neck deformity; Rheumatoid arthritis

1. Causes of swan neck deformity

Zancolli [1] proposed a classification of the types of swan neck deformity according to the initiating pathology (Table 1).

1.1. Pathomechanics

Weakness of the PIP joint stabilising mechanisms and increased power of the long extensors and intrinsic muscles cause hyperextension of the PIP joint and dorsomedial dislocation of the lateral bands of the extensor tendons (Table 2). The changing geometry of the extensor apparatus elongates the lateral bands and shortens the proximal extensor, causing drooping of the DIP joint and further hyperextension at the PIP joint. The oblique retinacular ligament shifts so that it passes dorsal to the axis of the PIP joint and a progressively worsening deformity occurs.

E-mail address: simon.knight@leedsth.nhs.uk.

0531-5131/ © 2006 Published by Elsevier B.V.
doi:10.1016/j.ics.2006.03.066

Table 1
Zancolli classification of the causes of swan neck deformity

Type of swan neck deformity	Pathology	Causes
Extrinsic	Increased power of traction of the long extensor tendon	Flexed positions of wrist or MCP joints Mallet deformity
Intrinsic	Increased power of traction of the intrinsic muscles	Intrinsic tightness secondary to MCP joint subluxation
Articular	Weakening of PIP joint stabilising mechanisms	Volar plate insufficiency FDS insufficiency Failure of transverse retinacular ligament of Landsmeer

1.2. Examination

Assessment of the deformity involves examination to try to determine the causes of the deformity (Table 1: articular, extrinsic, intrinsic) and to assess the flexibility and radiological state of the PIP joint.

Intrinsic tightness is diagnosed with the Finochietto-Bunnell test: When the proximal phalanx is held in extension at the MCP joint, the distal phalanges cannot be flexed; flexion of the MCP joint allows flexion of the distal phalanges.

Assessment of the fingers allows them to be classified into four clinical groups as suggested by Nalebuff [2] (Table 3).

2. Treatment

The treatment depends on the clinical group (Table 4).

Flexor synovectomy. This should be considered early. Synovectomy of the PIP joint may be required as well.

FDS sling [3]. This is a simple and effective method of correcting the hyperextension deformity at the PIP joint. It may be performed at the same time as a flexor synovectomy. The ulnar slip of the FDS is divided proximal to the decussation. It is left attached at its

Table 2
Pathomechanics of swan neck deformity (after Zancolli)

Cause of the deformity	Weakening of PIP joint stabilization mechanisms Increased power of traction of the intrinsic muscles Increased power of traction of long extensors
First pathologic stage	PIP joint recurvatum Dorsomedial dislocation of the conjoint lateral extensor tendons
Second pathologic stage	Dysfunction of the extensor apparatus by asymmetry (relative lengthening of the lateral bands and relative shortening of the proximal conjoint extensor tendon) Increase of extension force over middle phalanx leading to progressive recurvatum of the PIP joint Reduction of extension force over the distal phalanx leading to progressive flexion of the distal joint

Table 3
Nalebuff clinical classification of swan neck deformity

Type	Characteristics
Type 1	Full range of motion, no intrinsic tightness, no functional limitations
Type 2	Intrinsic tightness
	Limited PIP joint motion with extended MCP joint with ulnar deviation corrected
Type 3	Stiff PIP joint in all positions of the MCP joint
	X ray shows well preserved joint space
Type 4	Stiff PIP joint with destruction of joint surfaces

insertion and its proximal end is passed through a loop in the distal end of the A2 pulley and sutured on itself to create a strong check to full extension of the PIP joint. If the A2 pulley is of poor quality, the slip can be attached to the bone of the proximal phalanx.

Dermodesis involves excising an ellipse of skin from the flexor surface of the finger over the PIP joint. It often re stretches and is only suitable for mild deformities of the PIP joint and is often used in conjunction with fusion of the distal interphalangeal joint.

Distal joint fusion. When the primary lesion is a mallet deformity and there is radiological evidence of distal joint destruction, arthrodesis is the treatment of choice. This may be performed in conjunction with a dermodesis of the PIP joint.

Oblique retinacular ligament reconstruction [4]. This reconstruction was first suggested by Littler. It prevents hyper extension of the proximal interphalangeal joint while extending the distal joint. The classic reconstruction involves dividing the ulnar lateral extensor tendon at the musculotendinous junction at the base of the proximal phalanx. The band is dissected to its insertion and rerouted volar to Cleland's ligament. It is secured to the proximal flexor sheath at the A2 pulley. For a more secure repair, the lateral band may be routed across the palmar surface of the PIP joint and secured to the bone of the radial side of the proximal phalanx. A modification of this technique uses the uses a tendon graft [5] instead of the lateral band, if the lateral band is of poor quality.

Table 4
Options for the surgical treatment of swan neck deformity according to the nalebuff clinical classification

Type	MCP joint	PIP joint	DIP joint
Type 1		Dermodesis	Fusion
		Flexor synovectomy	
		FDS sling	
		Littler oblique retinacular ligament reconstruction	
		Zancolli lateral band translocation	
Type 2	Intrinsic release		
	MCP joint replacement if needed		
Type3		PIP joint manipulation	
		Skin release	
		Lateral band mobilisation	
Type 4		Arthrodesis (especially index and middle)	
		Arthroplasty(especially middle and little)	

Zancolli lateral band translocation. In this procedure, the lateral extensor tendon on the radial side of the finger is raised. In contrast to the oblique retinacular ligament reconstruction, the proximal part of the tendon is not divided and the tendon is raised as a bucket handle. The tendon is then subluxed volarwards and is maintained in this position by placing it deep to a sling made by suturing the volar plate to the FDS. This technique gives good and predictable results [6].

Littler's Intrinsic release [7]. When the clinical tests demonstrate intrinsic tightness in the presence of MCP joint deformity, an MCP joint arthroplasty, with adequate bony resection and ulnar intrinsic release will deal with the problem. In patients without MCP joint subluxation, resection of the oblique fibres of the intrinsic hood restores the ability to flex the distal phalanges when the MCP joint held in extension.

PIP joint manipulation and lateral band mobilisation [8]. This may be useful in those cases with limitation of PIP joint motion, where there is radiological evidence of a reasonable PIP joint. The fingers are passively flexed. When the deformity cannot be corrected by manipulation, the dorsum of the finger is opened through a curved incision and the lateral bands are surgically separated from the central tendon. The joint is the re manipulated and the lateral bands gently sublux laterally and volarwards as the finger flexes. The correction is maintained with a K wire. The dorsal skin may be too tight to completely close and part of the wound may have to be left open.

Arthrodesis. When the PIP joint is destroyed, most rewarding procedure is an arthrodesis. In the index and middle fingers, this should be in a position that restores precision grip.

Arthroplasty. The little and ring fingers, by contrast, require a reasonable range of motion for a good power grip. An arthroplasty is the preferred option.

References

[1] E.A. Zancolli, Structural and Dynamic Bases of Hand Surgery, 2nd ed., JB Lippincott Company, Philadelphia, 1979.

[2] E.A. Nalebuff, The rheumatoid swan neck deformity, Hand Clin. 5 (1989) 203–214.

[3] R. Curtis, Sublimis tenodesis, Campbell's Operative Othopaedics, 6th ed, The CV Mosby Co, St Louis, 1980, 319 pp.

[4] J.W. Littler, Restoration of the oblique retinacular ligament for correcting hyperextension deformity of the proximal interphalangeal joint, La Main Rheumatismale, L'Expansion Scientifique Francaise, Paris, 1966, pp. 39–42.

[5] J.S. Thompson, J.W. Littler, J. Upton, The spiral oblique retinacular ligament (SORL), J. Hand Surg. 3 (1978) 482–487.

[6] M.A. Tonkin, J. Hughes, K.L. Smith, Lateral band translocation for swan neck deformity, J. Hand Surg. 17A (1992) 260–267.

[7] J.W. Littler, Referred to in D.C. Riordan, C. Harris. Intrinsic contracture in the hand and its surgical treatment. J. Bone Jt. Surg. 36A (1954) 10–20.

[8] B.J. Gainor, G.L. Hummel, Correction of rheumatoid swan neck deformity by lateral band mobilisation, J. Hand Surg. 10A (1985) 370–376.

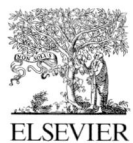

International Congress Series 1295 (2006) 158–161

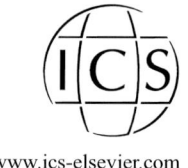

www.ics-elsevier.com

PIP joint surgery in rheumatoid disease

R.D. Beckenbaugh

Mayo Clinic, Department of Orthopedic Surgery, 200 First St., SW, Rochester, MN 55905, United States

Abstract. The proximal interphalangeal (PIP) joint in rheumatoid arthritis is often involved with disabling pain and deformity. Correction of swan-neck deformity is easier than correction of boutonniere deformity. Total joint arthroplasty is now available and is capable of treating most PIP disease in rheumatoid arthritis. However if the metacarpophalangeal (MCP) joints are involved, fusion of the PIP is more often appropriate. © 2006 Elsevier B.V. All rights reserved.

Keywords: Rheumatoid arthritis; Swan-neck; Boutonniere; PIP total joint arthroplasty

The PIP joint in rheumatoid arthritis may be involved in many deformities. These are intimately related to disease status of the wrist and MCP and occasionally to disease at the DIP. As with any joint in rheumatoid arthritis, synovitis leads to joint instability secondary to distension of soft tissues as well as destruction of bony architecture through cartilage wear and bony erosions.

The classic deformities of the PIP in RA are swan-neck, boutonniere and ulnar deviation.

Swan-neck deformity develops in the presence of intrinsic tightness or extrinsic imbalance (associated with loss of carpal height) [3]. MCP joint stability is directly related to swan-neck deformity. If the MCP joint subluxes decompression of the intrinsic forces usually prevents swan-neck deformity. Another frequently missed but important contributor to swan-neck deformity is flexor tenosynovitis with adherence of the superficialis tendon in the A-1 and A-2 pulley areas resulting in an ineffective flexor force at the PIP [1].

Boutonniere deformity develops from synovitic attenuation of the central slip and/or retinacular membrane supporting the lateral bands. While the MCP status has an effect on the forces leading to the boutonniere deformity, the intrinsic disease at the PIP joint itself is

E-mail address: beckenbaugh.robert@mayo.edu.

0531-5131/ © 2006 Elsevier B.V. All rights reserved.
doi:10.1016/j.ics.2006.03.023

the major reason for this deformity (not effected by wrist or MCP status as compared to swan-neck).

Ulnar deviation deformity is a secondary phenomenon that occurs from ulnarly direct forces applied to the unstable PIP (pinch). It generally occurs with very proliferate joint synovitis and an MCP joint which remains longitudinally oriented. Ulnar deviation and instability is functionally very disabling.

The baseline treatment for advanced rheumatoid disease of the PIP joint is arthrodesis. This operation is simple to do and effective in improving function with a low failure rate. In the presence of significant MCP disease with the need for arthroplasty, PIP arthroplasty is generally not indicated as rehabilitation of both joints is very difficult. On the other hand, PIP fusion enhances the results of MCP arthroplasty by concentrating the tendon forces at that joint.

In early swan-neck deformity with intact articular contour, soft tissue procedures may be very helpful in correcting the deformity. If the MCP is subluxed this must be addressed first or at the same time as swan-neck corrective surgery. First, the status of the superficialis must be known and through a dorsal MCP arthroplasty exposure or through a volar proximal phalangeal oblique exposure they are pulled and/or "freed" to assure their functional excursion. Two basic methods of management are then available to correct the deformity. The first is simple and involves release of the dorsally displaced lateral bands +/ − the extensor tendon (by tenotomy) and suture of the lateral bands volarly to the collateral ligaments or volar retinacular membranes. The "Matev" procedure releases one central tendon and allows the other to transfer volarly to provide DIP extension [4]. Simple volar transfer of the lateral bands may be sufficient in mild "swan-necking". In more severe deformities (>20° hyperextension), a more stable form of correction is superficialis hemitenodesis. This can be accomplished by splitting the decussation and incising the ulnar half of the superficialis proximally. The distally attached tendon strip is then passed as a loop through the distal one-third of the A-2 pulley and sutured back to itself with a non-absorbable suture. The tenodesis is tied with the PIP in 15°–20° of flexion and immediate postoperative motion is allowed [1].

Correction of boutonniere deformity in rheumatoid arthritis is difficult. In my experience, advancement or imbrication of the central tendon is seldom successful. The Littler–Eaton rollover of the lateral bands, bringing them dorsally and suturing them to each other is often more effective [2]. In the majority of RA patients with boutonniere deformity, arthrodesis is preferred. The DIP joint may require extensor release.

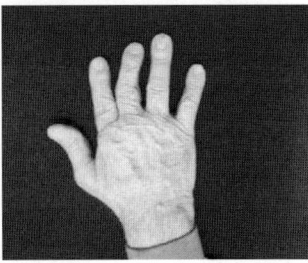

Fig. 1. Patient with ulnar deviation through PIP.

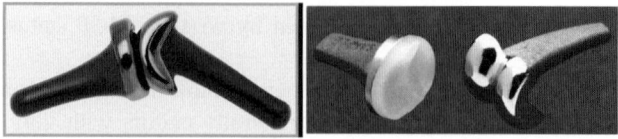

Fig. 2. SBI SR PIP implant (right), Ascension "Pyrocarbon" implant (left).

In ulnar deviation deformity arthrodesis is preferred although new solid-type of joint implants may allow correction of this deformity with maintenance of motion. Silicone arthroplasty is not indicated in this type of deformity as recurrent ulnar deviation deformity will almost always occur (Fig. 1).

Arthroplasty of the PIP joint is now a realistic option in patients with RA. Past experiences with silicone devices have been disappointing with gradual subsidence and loss of motion, fracture of implant with swelling and recurrent deformity all being common. Early experience with the solid fixed fulcrum implants, reconstruction as opposed to arthrodesis appears to be a reasonable option.

In the U.S., currently the SBI SR resurfacing and the Ascension "Pyrocarbon" implants are available as FDA Humanitarian device exemption implants (Fig. 2).

These devices will assist in reconstruction of stiff, hyperextended and angulated (ulnar deviation) deformities in RA. Boutonniere deformities, however, remain a challenge of reconstruction with implants because of deficient central extensor tendons.

My greatest experience in PIP arthroplasty is with the pyrocarbon device. Correction of swan-neck deformities and ulnar deviation deformities is relatively easy to achieve with

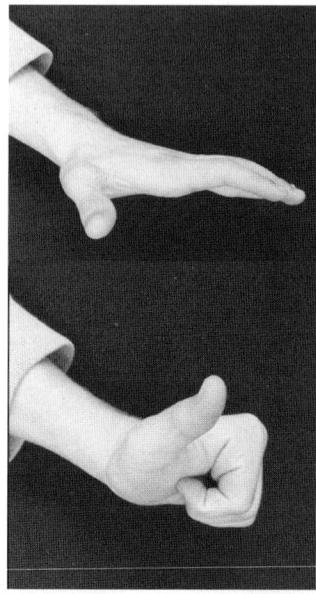

Fig. 3. Patient with arthroplasty for PIP disease. Motion postop superficialis hemitenodesis performed for swan-neck deformity.

these PIP solid implants. The patients with painful synovitis and joint destruction without deformity are also good candidates. The presence of excess instability in multiple directions as seen in "loose" type of RA and arthritis mutilans may be followed by implant instability and these patients are best served by arthrodesis. The implants are inserted through a dorsal extensor splitting approach. Using saw guides, broaches and burrs, the joint surfaces are prepared for insertion of the stemmed nonhinged implants. The pyrocarbon implants have a small amount of "slop" in the articulation to provide for mobilization and strain reduction. The metal and polyethylene device is a close fixed articulation and may be inserted with or without cement although removal of a cemented implant can be very difficult.

Pain relief is generally excellent and approximated 60° of motion is achieved. Fig. 3 shows a good clinical result 3.5 years postop correction of PIP disease of the index and long finger in a 54-year-old patient. Superficialis hemitenodesis was performed as a secondary procedure in this patient who is pain free and very happy with the result (Fig. 3).

Surgical treatment of the PIP joint in RA includes soft tissue rebalancing, arthrodesis, and arthroplasty. In most instances, if MCP disease is present, the PIP joint should be arthrodesed. In situations with located functioning MCP joints, arthroplasty may be appropriate.

References

[1] F.D. Beckenbaugh, Superficialis tenodesis to the A-2 pulley for swan-neck deformity in rheumatoid arthritis, Orthop. Trans. 8 (1984) 382.
[2] J.W. Littler, R.G. Eaton, Redistribution of forces in the correction of boutonniere deformity, J. Bone Joint Surg 49A (7) (1967) 1267–1274.
[3] J. Shapiro, J.S. Shapiro, Wrist involvement in rheumatoid swan-neck deformity, J Hand Surg 7A (5) (1982) 484–491.
[4] R.Q. Terrill, R.J. Groves, Correction of the severe nonrheumatoid chronic boutonniere deformity with a modified Matev procedure, J Hand Surg 17A (5) (1992) 874–880.

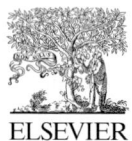

International Congress Series 1295 (2006) 162–168

ELSEVIER

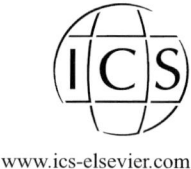

www.ics-elsevier.com

Classification and treatment of the rheumatoid thumb

Matthew M. Tomaino *

Division of Hand, Shoulder, and Elbow Surgery, University of Rochester Medical Center, Rochester, NY, USA
Hand and Upper Extremity Fellowship, University of Rochester Medical Center, Rochester, NY, USA

Abstract. The rheumatoid thumb is amenable to satisfactory surgical treatment. An understanding of the classification of deformity facilitates selection of optimal treatment strategy. © 2006 Published by Elsevier B.V.

Keywords: Rheumatoid thumb deformity; Surgical treatment

Thumb deformities are present in 60% to 81% of patients with rheumatoid arthritis. These deformities may lead to significant impairment in hand function because the thumb accounts for approximately 40–50% of hand function. Impaired function of the thumb may be caused by abnormalities in the joints, musculotendinous units, and neurologic structures. When determining appropriate treatment for the rheumatoid thumb, therefore, all extrinsic (soft tissue) as well as intrinsic (bone and joint) factors contributing to thumb function must be assessed. This review will address classification and treatment of thumb deformity.

1. Classification of thumb deformity

Rheumatoid arthritis may involve all joints of the thumb. Because the function of each joint is closely linked, involvement or deformity of one joint may eventually lead to a predictable deformity of the others. Nalebuff introduced a classification of common deformities of the rheumatoid thumb in 1968. Subsequently, other categories have been added. The classification encompasses the majority of thumb deformities, but is not all-inclusive. As might be expected, thumb deformity caused by arthritis presents in hands with other problems as well, including wrist and finger deformity or arthritis.

* 601 Elmwood Avenue Box 665, Rochester, NY 14642, USA. Tel.: +1 585 273 3157.
E-mail address: matthew_tomaino@urmc.rochester.edu.

0531-5131/ © 2006 Published by Elsevier B.V.
doi:10.1016/j.ics.2006.03.009

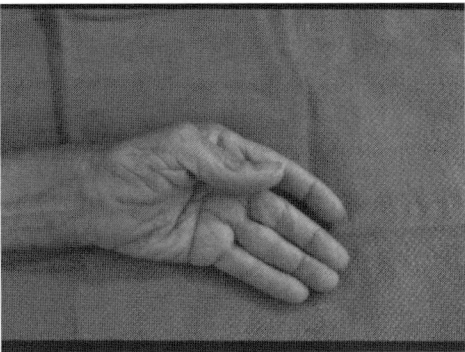

Fig. 1. Type I deformity. a. Preoperative picture.

The type I deformity or boutonniere deformity is the most commonly seen when treating the rheumatoid patient (Fig. 1). An awareness of the pathogenesis of this deformity explains why the MP joint is the one most commonly affected in the rheumatoid thumb. The deformity typically begins with MCP joint synovitis. With capsular distention, the extensor mechanism becomes involved and slowly attenuates at the extensor pollicis brevis (EPB) insertion. A lag develops as the extensor hood becomes incompetent; the EPL tendon subluxates ulnarly and moves volar to the center of rotation of the joint. This increases the flexion deformity. The IP joint becomes hyperextended secondary to increased forces on the distal phalanx from the intrinsics and EPL. The first metacarpal typically assumes an abducted position to compensate for the flexion deformity of the MCP joint. Ultimately, this deformity becomes fixed and if longstanding, volar subluxation or frank dislocation of the proximal phalanx may result in bony erosion on its dorsal proximal aspect (Fig. 2).

Other causes of type I deformity exist, but are not as common. A similar deformity may occur following rupture of the EPL or FPL tendons. Rupture of the EPL leads to MP joint deformity because of the inability of the brevis to fully extend the MP joint by itself. In cases in which the FPL ruptures, IP joint hyperextension deformity occurs if the volar plate becomes incompetent. The MCP joint flexion deformity is secondary. Nalebuff believed this deformity was better termed an *extrinsic minus deformity*, because the cause is usually secondary to an incompetent or ruptured extrinsic tendon to the thumb. In assessing any type I deformity, therefore, all extrinsic tendons should be assessed individually.

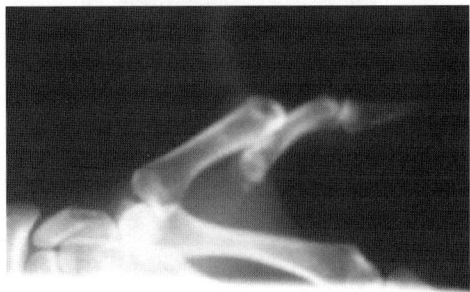

Fig. 2. Radiograph of a chronic type I thumb deformity.

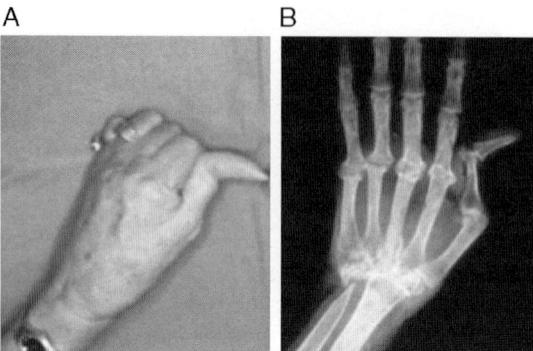

Fig. 3. Type II deformity. A. Preoperative picture. B. Preoperative X-ray.

The remaining categories in Nalebuff's *original* description, type II and type III deformities, stem from initial pathology at the trapeziometacarpal (TM) joint. Type II deformity is rarely encountered and, in 1984, Nalebuff recommended its removal from the classification system. Its inclusion in the system, however, has persisted. In type II deformity, the TM joint subluxates, leading to metacarpal adduction, MCP flexion, and IP extension (Fig. 3). Its importance in the classification is to differentiate it from type I deformity, in which the TM joint is not involved. Although type I and II thumbs may appear alike clinically, therefore, the TM joint requires treatment in the latter.

Type III is the second most common deformity and is termed a *swan-neck deformity* (Fig. 4). Initial pathology occurs at the TM joint. Synovitis leads to capsular laxity and dorsoradial subluxation of the metacarpal base. The metacarpal shaft assumes an adducted position. Secondary extensor imbalance and subsequent volar plate laxity of the MCP joint lead to a hyperextension deformity of the joint and, occasionally, secondary IP joint flexion.

Type IV and type V deformities begin at the MCP joint. Synovitis of the joint leads to laxity of the ulnar collateral ligament or the volar plate, respectively. Type IV deformity,

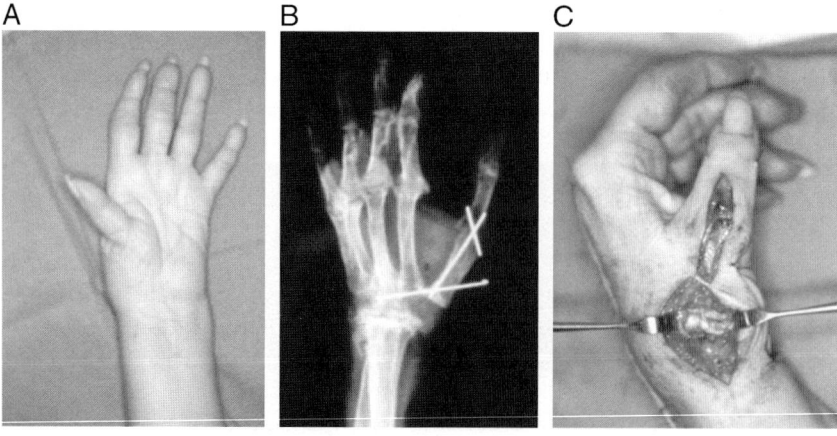

Fig. 4. Type III deformity. A. Preoperative picture. B. Postoperative X-ray after trapezium resection and suspensionplasty. C. Intraoperative picture of the EPB suspensionplasty.

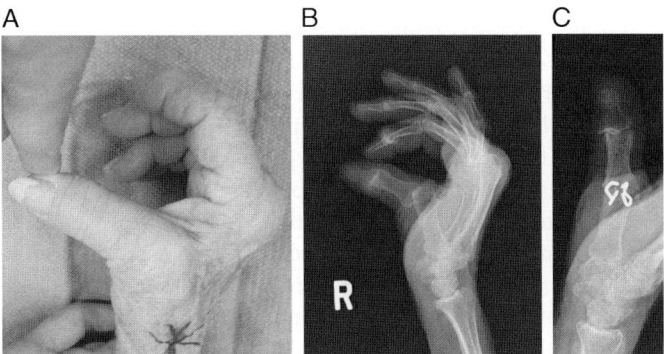

Fig. 5. Type IV deformity. A. Preoperative picture of a type IV deformity. B. Preoperative X-ray. C. Postoperative X-ray following fusion.

which is more common than type V, is also termed *gamekeeper's deformity* (Fig. 5). Valgus deformity causes subsequent adduction of the metacarpal. The first web space, adductor pollicis and first dorsal interosseous muscle may become contracted. Type V deformity results from attenuation of the volar plate of the MCP joint, and leads to an isolated hyperextension deformity. A flexion deformity of the IP joint ensues secondary to tendon imbalance. The TM joint is not involved in type IV or type V deformities. Type VI deformity results from gross bony destruction, and leads to significant instability and subsequent shortening. This deformity, termed *arthritis mutilans*, may lead to any type of deformity of the MCP or IP joints.

The more common thumb deformities tend to lead to reciprocal deformities of adjacent joints. Such reciprocal deformity is characteristic of the longitudinal intercalated collapse deformity seen in the osteoarthritic thumb with TM arthritis and MP hyperextension deformity. These deformities are accentuated by tendon imbalance and use of the thumb during lateral pinch. The deformities initially are flexible, but may become fixed if ignored.

2. Treatment of thumb deformity

The goals of treatment of the rheumatoid thumb include pain relief, prevention or correction of deformity, and improvement in function. A pain-free, stable thumb is the overall objective. Stability is more important than improving motion, particularly at the IP and MP joints. In that light, maintaining motion at the TM joint is advantageous. Fundamentally, this provides a mobile post for pinch and prehension. Though postoperative strength and function will not be normal, patient satisfaction is frequently improved.

Not all patients with deformity of the thumb require reconstruction. There are cases, however, in which severe deformity, alone, even without symptoms, may best be treated. In type I thumbs that are dislocated or subluxed, for example, erosion of the proximal dorsal surface of the proximal phalanx by the metacarpal head may complicate arthrodesis (Fig. 2).

In other words, while surgical correction of deformity assumes that a patient experiences pain or functional impairment, even in the absence thereof, surgical intervention is warranted in certain situations where delay may jeopardize success in the future.

Other parts of the upper extremity must be assessed and treated prior to, or in association with, thumb reconstruction. Shoulder and elbow abnormalities are usually addressed first so their diminished function does not impede hand rehabilitation. Neurologic deficits, such as carpal tunnel syndrome, and wrist pathology should be corrected prior to, or at the time of, thumb surgery. Deformity of other digits may take precedence over the thumb, depending on the patient's functional requirements and pain level. It must be remembered, however, that results are typically better when reconstruction is performed prior to development of advanced disease, and there is no more successful an operation, in the rheumatoid patient, than thumb MCP joint fusion. Accordingly, favorable outcome following thumb reconstruction can improve a patient's overall attitude about and confidence in subsequent surgeries. Additionally, the patient must be aware that rheumatoid arthritis may be a progressive disease, and the result of surgery may diminish with time. If painful symptoms persist despite medical management for 4 to 6 months, function is significantly impaired by deformity, or advanced joint destruction is noted, surgical reconstruction is indicated.

3. Treatment of the metacarpophalangeal joint

The MP joint is most commonly affected by deformity and therefore is the most likely to require surgery. In correcting deformity, incompetent or ruptured tendons and ligaments must be addressed as well as the tendon imbalance.

Nalebuff described "EPL rerouting" as a procedure to treat early type I deformities. The EPL tendon is passed through the dorsal capsule at the base of the proximal phalanx and sutured to itself. The EPB is sutured to the longus and the extensor hood is advanced. The thumb intrinsic muscles provide for IP joint extension. A high recurrence rate may complicate this procedure. An alternative procedure reattaches the EPB to the base of the proximal phalanx through capsule or bone. The EPL is stabilized dorsally, reconstructing the extensor hood. Inglis has desribed suturing the abductor pollicis brevis and adductor pollicis to the EPL tendon to keep the tendon centralized. Secondary instability of the MP joint may recur, however, as with any soft tissue procedure. Subsequent pain or deformity may occur at the IP or TM joints, but less frequently than after MCP arthrodesis. In that light, the author prefers to treat type I thumb deformities with arthrodesis. Thumb MP joint arthrodesis is reliable and provides excellent function. Soft tissue procedures at the MCP joint for type III, IV, and V deformities are aimed at correcting the hyperextension or valgus deformity. Though soft tissue procedures are an option, I routinely recommend arthrodesis.

The primary goal of treatment is pain relief and stability. Long-term results of arthrodesis are favorable. Fusion rates vary between 83% and 100%. Nalebuff has recommended that arthrodesis he performed in 15° flexion, 20° pronation, and 5° abduction. Techniques for arthrodesis include crossed Kirschner wires, tension-band techniques, the use of Herbert screws, and staples. All produce similar results. I prefer either k-wires or staples. Interphalangeal motion should be initiated as soon as possible to prevent tendon adherence at the fusion site. In cases of arthritis mutilans, cancellous bone graft or bone blocks may be required. In these cases, time for complete fusion may be prolonged and immobilization should be adjusted appropriately.

For type I deformities, options also include arthroplasty. Collateral ligament stability is mandatory for arthroplasty. If the collateral ligaments do not provide adequate stability or

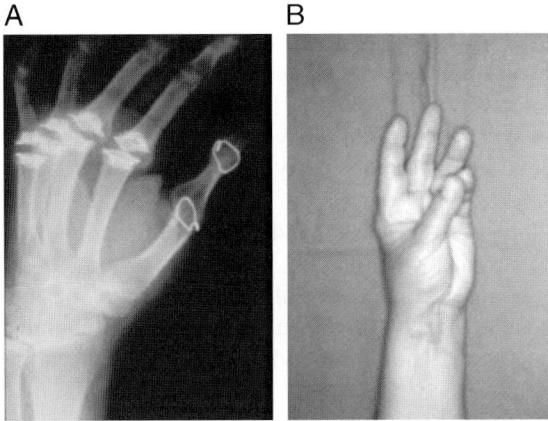

Fig. 6. Sequential MP and IP joint fusion. a. Postoperative X-ray. b. Postoperative picture.

cannot be reconstructed, arthrodesis should be performed. Arthroplasty is indicated in older patients and in thumbs with significant IP or TM joint involvement. Theoretically, it is preferable to avoid arthrodesis of both the IP and MCP joints. If IP joint fusion is required, consideration should be given to MCP arthroplasy. The author has little experience with MCP joint arthroplasty, however, and has noted satisfactory function following combined MCP and IP joint fusion when a mobile TM joint is present or reconstructed (Fig. 6). Greater than 90% of patients undergoing MP arthroplasties achieve good to excellent results. Nevertheless, one can expect superb function without risk of recurrent deformity when arthrodesis is selected.

4. Interphalangeal joint

Dysfunction at the IP joint may result from tendon rupture. Treatment options depend on the stability of the joint and the quality of the articular surface. Alternatives for treatment of IP joint deformity secondary to synovitis or tendon imbalance include synovectomy, Kirschner-wire fixation, joint release, hemitenodesis, and arthrodesis. Arthroplasy is not indicated. Synovectomy is indicated when synovitis has been present for 4–6 months despite medical therapy or, occasionally, when the joint is symptomatic and concomitant surgery is being performed on the hand.

Treatment of joint hyperextension associated with type I deformity has included pinning of the joint in flexion when deformity can be corrected, passively, and a dorsal joint release if the deformity is fixed. Both have been noted to have a high incidence of recurrence when MCP joint reconstruction is being performed. If the articular surface is of good quality, I recommend that the hyperextension deformity be treated with a Krischner wire in slight flexion for 4 weeks. If the deformity is fixed or significant collateral instability is noted, arthrodesis is preferred. As has been noted, I do not regard MP joint fusion for the type I thumb as a contraindication to IP joint fusion in cases when rigid hyperextension requires release and stabilization.

5. Trapeziometacarpal joint

Treatment of TM joint pathology is directed at relieving pain, restoring stability, and maintaining motion. Arthrodesis of the TM joint is not advisable, particularly in light of the likelihood that the MP and IP joints may require arthrodesis at some time. Resection arthroplasty and silicone implant arthroplasty are options in older patients with extremely low-demand thumbs.

I no longer use implant arthroplasty and rely on trapezium resection and ligament reconstruction/suspensionplasty. For type II and III thumbs, I always perform a suspensionplasty as opposed to excisional arthroplasty alone to avoid the risk of instability and scaphometacarpal impingement—a more likely complication after this latter procedure in the rheumatoid thumb, in which the intermetacarpal ligament is often attenuated.

Although the flexor carpi radialis tendon can be used to suspend the base of the thumb, I selectively use the EPB tendon. In most symptomatic type II and III thumbs, MP joint arthrodesis is performed at the same time. In these cases, the EPB tendon is a very feasible donor tendon. The EPB is released at its myotendinous junction and passed either through the dorsum of the metacarpal, out through its base in the plane of the nail–or through the capsule without using a bony channel–and then around the FCR to create a suspension sling (Fig. 4). Alternatively the EPB tendon can be attached to the radial aspect of the index metacarpal base with a suture anchor.

6. Summary

Rheumatoid arthritis commonly affects the thumb. Deformity does not require surgical intervention unless pain is present or a functional deficit exits, but if bony erosion develops and surgical treatment may be compromised in the future, earlier intervention may be indicated. When the pathogenesis and pathoanatomy of the impaired rheumatoid thumb are appreciated, and appropriate treatment is selected, surgical intervention is likely to provide a favorable outcome for the patient.

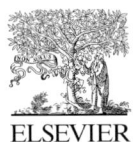

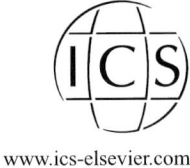

www.ics-elsevier.com

Is there a role for silicone trapezial replacement in the rheumatoid hand?

Alberto Lluch *

Institut Kaplan, Paseo Bonanova, 9, 08022 Barcelona, Spain

Abstract. Destruction of the T-MC joint can be treated by arthrodesis or arthroplasty. Arthrodesis is not recommended because it requires a long period of immobilization, which is not well tolerated by the rheumatoid patient. Furthermore, it will increase the forces at the metacarpophalangeal and interphalangeal joints, increasing their deformities. Trapezoidectomy, with or without tendon interposition and ligament reconstruction, is usually recommended but may cause some basal thumb instability and prolonged postoperative discomfort. Replacement of the trapezium with a silicone implant restores length to the thumb ray, and postoperative recovery is much shorter. The main complication is implant dislocation, which can be prevented if the following is done: use the smallest size implant, create a concavity on the trapezoid bone and stabilize the implant with a slip of the *flexor carpi radialis* tendon carefully sutured to the distal scaphoid capsule. Transfixing the body of the implant with a Kirschner wire ensures implant stabilization during capsular healing and allows immediate postoperative mobility of the thumb. © 2006 Elsevier B.V. All rights reserved.

Keywords: Rheumatoid thumb; Trapezio-metacarpal joint arthroplasty; Silicone implant

1. Rheumatoid thumb deformities

Rheumatoid thumb deformities can be secondary to tendon ruptures, joint synovitis or both. Synovitis of the trapezio-metacarpal (T-MC) joint will cause a dorso-radial dislocation of the metacarpal, resulting in an adduction T-MC joint deformity, a secondary hyperextension deformity of the metacarpophalangeal (MP) joint and flexion of the interphalangeal (IP) joint. This is the type III thumb deformity described by Nalebuff [1], resembling the swan-neck collapse deformity seen in the three-phalanx fingers (Fig. 1).

* Tel.: +34 93 417 84 84; fax: +34 93 211 04 02.
E-mail addresses: alluch@telefonica.net, albertolluch@infonegocio.com.

0531-5131/ © 2006 Elsevier B.V. All rights reserved.
doi:10.1016/j.ics.2006.03.072

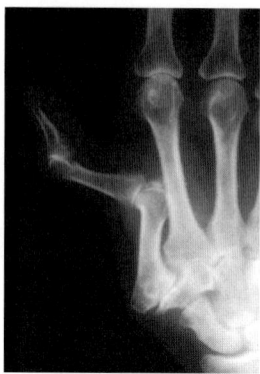

Fig. 1. Swan-neck or type III deformity, according to Nalebuff's classification.

Synovitis of the metacarpophalangeal joint will attenuate the dorsal capsular and tendon structures, causing a flexion deformity of the joint and a hyperextension deformity of the interphalangeal joint. This is the type I deformity described by Nalebuff [1], similar to a boutonnière deformity of the three-phalanx fingers. When the collateral ligaments are weakened by the synovitis, a lateral instability will also occur, corresponding to the type IV deformity.

The MP joint is frequently the first to show signs of rheumatoid arthritis in the hand. Synovitis is also probably present in other joints of the hand, particularly the MP joints of the three-phalanx fingers, but the work demands on the thumb MP joint are so great that functional deterioration first shows up here [2]. In the presence of a flexion deformity of the MP joint, the patient will keep the thumb metacarpal in abduction to hold and manipulate objects and, in later stages, in order to keep the thumb tip away from the flexion arch of the fingers. When the thumb metacarpal is abducted, the T-MC joint becomes more stable, and therefore "protected" from the deleterious effects of joint synovitis at this level (Fig. 2). For this reason, patients with rheumatoid arthritis present a lesser incidence of T-MC joint arthritis than women in the same age group who are free of rheumatoid disease.

Nalebuff has frequently expressed his regret at including the original type II deformity, which rarely occurs and is now recognized as being a combination of features of the original types I (MP joint synovitis) and III (T-MC joint synovitis) [3].

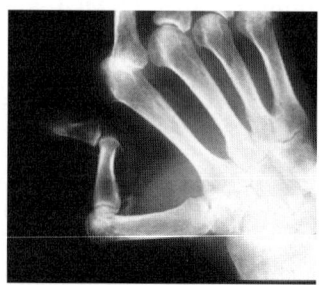

Fig. 2. Boutonnière or type I deformity according to Nalebuff's classification.

2. Treatment options for trapezio-metacarpal joint arthritis

When the T-MC joint has been destroyed, only arthrodesis or arthroplasty are the treatments of choice. Arthrodesis is not usually recommended in the rheumatoid thumb, not only because of an important functional loss but mainly because it has been proven to increase the forces at the distal joints, thus increasing their deformities.

Three different types of arthroplasty can be considered: excisional artroplasty, silicone implant arthroplasty and total joint arthroplasty. Total T-MC joint arthroplasty may be contraindicated in the rheumatoid patient, not only for having weak capsular tissue causing a higher rate of implant dislocation, but mainly due to poor bone stock. The trapezium has very little cortical bone and suffers from severe osteoporosis, increasing the incidence of component loosening or bone fracture. Often the trapezium is also deformed and flattened, and does not provide the necessary height to hold the proximal component of most total joint implants, which should be of about 8 mm.

Excisional arthroplasties, with or without tendon interposition, have been the most frequently procedures performed, although they cause thumb shortening and weakness. In order to decrease the magnitude of this complication, excisional arthroplasty has been associated with a ligament reconstruction and tendon interposition (LRTI) [4]. They usually require immobilization of the thumb in a position of abduction for 5 to 6 weeks to ensure good capsular healing [5].

Another alternative is the use of a silicone implant to replace the excised trapezium bone. Swanson silicone implant arthroplasty provides recovery of painless joint mobility within a short postoperative time [6,7].

3. Complications of silicone implants

The only complications which may occur are subluxation or dislocation of the implant [8–10] and possible foreign body reaction to silicone particles [9,11].

Foreign body reaction to silicone microparticles is referred to as "silicone synovitis". In general, the intensity of the reaction to microparticles depends upon the chemistry, size, number and, possibly, the shape of the particles [12]. The earlier theory of immunological response to silicone has been disproven. There is little or no evidence of immunological reactive cells; furthermore, silicone appears to be chemically inert and not enzymatically degraded by macrophages [13]. Because small particles are more likely to induce a greater inflammatory mediator release from macrophages than are larger particles, the trapezium and other spacer implants have been fabricated from "Conventional Silicone Elastomer" (CSE) since 1985. The wear debris from CSE is too large to be phagocytosed and is unimportant in the mechanism of particulate synovitis [13]. The incidence of silicone particulate synovitis is much lower in the trapezium than in any other carpal implants and very rare around flexible hinges [14,15].

The foreign body reaction to silicone particles observed with the use of lunate or scaphoid implants is secondary to the abrasion of its surface against the distal radius during wrist mobility. We performed fluoroscopic and dynamic radiographic examinations, on several patients in which a trapezium silicone implant was inserted, and it was demonstrated that thumb mobility took place at the stem of the implant, rather than at the interface between the implant and the scaphoid, thus explaining the absence of foreign body reaction to silicone particles.

Pellegrini and Burton [9] also described signs of deterioration of the implant in non-rheumatoid, with up to 50% wear of the vertical height at the ulnar margin, despite a very positive patient satisfaction rate.

We have done several biomechanical studies on the implant, including its placing under 1 million cycles of compression, with a frequency of 8 Hz, from 20 to 200 N, and no rupture or cold deformity were observed. The "cold flow" deformity observed by other authors is always secondary to wear of the implant, due to subluxation and friction against the distal scaphoid.

4. Surgical technique

A zigzag incision over the radial aspect of the wrist provides the best exposure and aesthetic result. The incision starts distally over the dorsum of the proximal third of the thumb metacarpal, and ends proximally just over the *flexor carpi radialis* (FCR) tendon about 3 cm proximal to the wrist flexion crease.

The sensory branches of the radial nerve should be identified and left undisturbed. After dividing the antebrachial fascia longitudinally, between the *abductor pollicis longus* (ABPL) tendon anteriorly and the *extensor pollicis brevis* (EPB) tendon posteriorly, the radial artery should be identified as it runs obliquely antero-proximally to dorso-distally. The approach to the base of the thumb metacarpal, the trapezium and distal end of the scaphoid is between the ABPL and EPB tendons. The periosteum and capsule are incised longitudinally and peeled off, anteriorly and posteriorly, from the base of the metacarpal and the trapezium until the scapho-trapezium (S-T) joint is identified. The capsule of the S-T joint should be detached very close to the trapezium in order to leave as much as possible attached to the scaphoid (Fig. 3).

The trapezium is fragmented and removed using a rongeur, until the tendon of the FCR is seen running in an oblique direction from the anterior aspect of the wrist (antero-

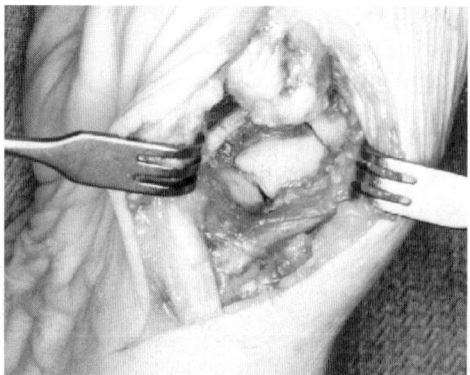

Fig. 3. After removal of the trapezium, the joint surfaces of the base of the index metacarpal, the trapezoid and the scaphoid can be visualized. Capsular attachments to the scaphoid have been preserved for later capsular reconstruction.

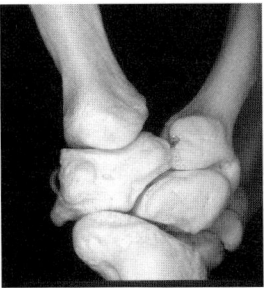

Fig. 4. The trapezium is a large bone, although the articular surface of the distal scaphoid, where the implant should be seated, is quite small. The joint surface of the trapezoid bone is convex.

proximal) to the base of the index metacarpal (dorso-distal). The portion of the trapezium that articulates with the trapezoid can easily be removed with the rongeur, but the rest of it is strongly attached to the thenar muscles, the flexor retinaculum and the intercarpal ligaments, and it should be removed using a sharp blade and cutting all structures very close to the bone. Any osteophyte or loose osteochondral body between the thumb and index metacarpals should also be removed. Using finger palpation, the anterior aspect of the base of the thumb metacarpal is explored and any bony prominence or osteophyte just distal to its anterior 'beak' is removed. The endomedullary bone of the thumb metacarpal is reamed with a rasp, creating a round endomedullary canal slightly larger than the triangular shaped stem of the implant, as we do not desire to create a "press-fit" stabilization or friction between the stem of the implant and bone. The base of the thumb metacarpal is then squared off, preserving the subchondral and cortical bone at the periphery as much as possible.

The trapezium is a large bone, although the articular surface of the distal scaphoid, where the implant should be seated, is quite small (Fig. 4). The exposed surface of the trapezoid is slightly convex and, by definition, two opposing convex surfaces are unstable; therefore, the implant will tend to displace to the dorsum. The proximal part of articular surface of the trapezoid with trapezium, just distal to the scaphoid joint, should

A   B

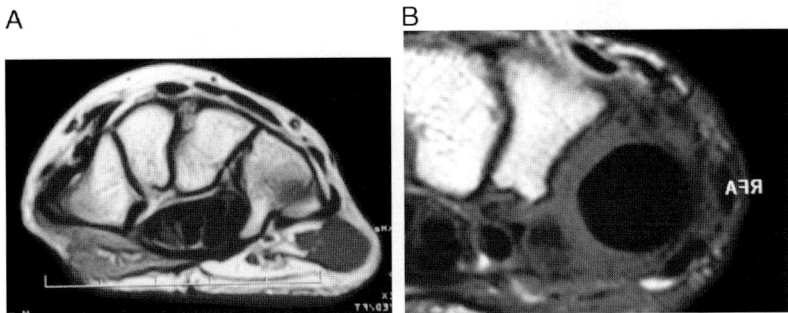

Fig. 5. (A) MRI examination of the distal carpal row bones, showing the slightly convex joint surface of the trapezoid bone with the trapezium. (B) MRI examination of a silicone trapezium implant, well-seated against the concavity created on the trapezoid.

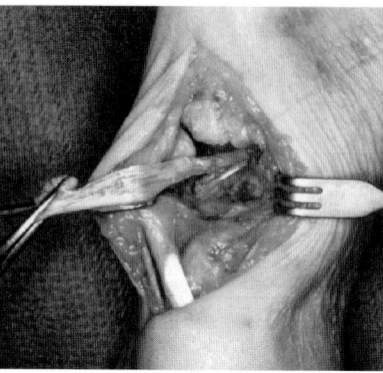

Fig. 6. A slip of the FCR tendon is passed from the distal forearm to the anterior facet of the trapezoid, preserving its distal insertion to the base of the index metacarpal.

be excised to make it slightly concave and provide more space and stability for the implant (Fig. 5A and B).

The antebrachial fascia is identified and through blunt dissection at the proximal end of the skin incision, it is incised longitudinally until the FCR tendon is visualized. Approximately 3 cm proximal to the wrist flexion crease, a slip of the FCR tendon comprising about three-quarters of its thickness is sectioned and later freed in a distal direction until its insertion into the base of the index metacarpal is reached. This division should be performed under direct vision to avoid rupture of the tendon. Previous incision of the compartment of the *flexor carpi radialis* will facilitate the passing of the tendon slip from the proximal to the distal aspect (Fig. 6).

A size 1 "Swanson"® silicone implant is then introduced into the medullary canal of the metacarpal to ensure full seating against the base of the metacarpal, and is later positioned exactly over the slightly convex articular surface of the scaphoid. The implant is secured in place with a fine Kirschner wire driven into the trapezoid (Fig. 7). Before introducing its stem into the metacarpal, it is easier to pierce the body of the implant transversely with the K-wire, which is left slightly protruding. This is done on the same sterile inner box in

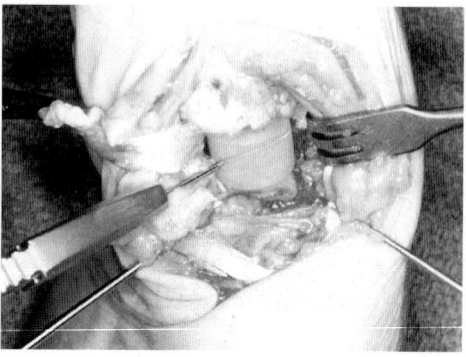

Fig. 7. The implant is placed over the distal scaphoid joint, and secured in place with a transfixing K-wire driven into the trapezoid.

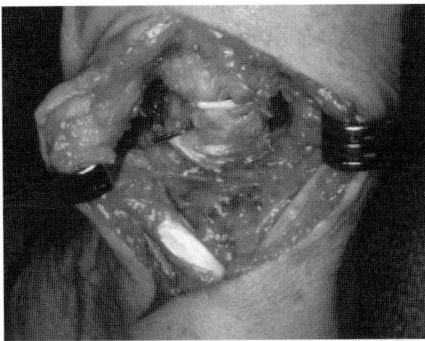

Fig. 8. The FCR tendon slip is carefully sutured to the distal scaphoid capsule, creating an annular ligament for implant stabilization.

which the implant is served by the manufacturer, thus avoiding the contact of the implant with surgical gauzes, as lint is easily attached to its surface and may cause a foreign body reaction. If the trapezoid convexity has been excavated, the K-wire will not slip anteriorly or posteriorly, and will easily penetrate the exposed cancellous bone. The K-wire should be directed almost in an anterior to dorsal direction in relation to the palm of the hand, and care should be taken to avoid placing the implant in a moderate dorsal displacement in relation to the distal scaphoid, as all of subluxations and dislocations occur dorsal to the scaphoid, mostly from improper initial positioning. The K-wire should then be cut about 5 mm over the surface of the implant.

The slip of the FRC tendon is pierced over the K-wire antero-dorsally in order to create an annular ligament, which will stabilize the implant. The proximal edge of the tendon slip is sutured to the capsule at the distal scaphoid with 1.5 metric (4–0 USP) PDS material, taking care not to injure the radial artery, which is now safely retracted (Fig. 8).

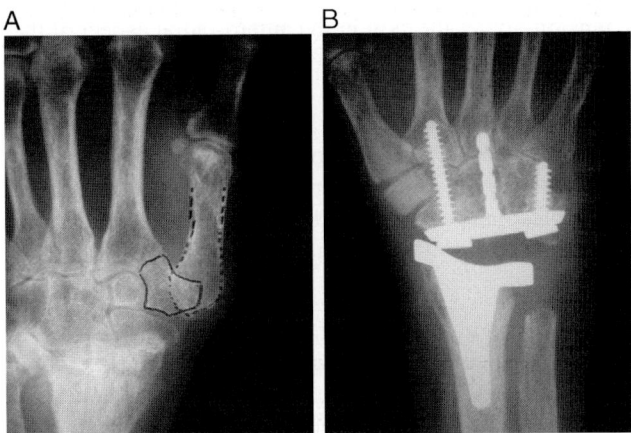

Fig. 9. (A) Complete T-MC joint dislocation and severe wrist joint destruction in a patient suffering from rheumatoid arthritis. (B) Even in cases of complete T-MC joint dislocation, the silicone implant will remain in place after annular capsular reconstruction with a broad slip of the FCR tendon.

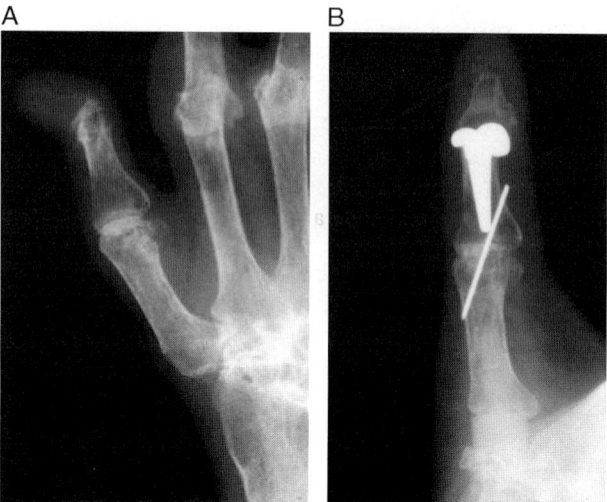

Fig. 10. (A) Radiograph of the thumb of a patient with MP joint instability and subluxation of both IP and T-MC joints. (B) The instability of the MP joint was treated by arthrodesis. Mobility of IP and T-MC joints is very important for adequate thumb function, and was treated by means of implant arthroplasties.

The capsular and periosteal tissues, previously incised longitudinally, are then sutured over the FCR tendon slip. Usually there is a redundancy of connective tissue in direct proportion to the degree of thumb metacarpal subluxation, which should preferably be plicated, or excised to avoid excessive bulkiness. The stability of the implant will depend mainly upon the tendon slip that has been sutured carefully to the scaphoid capsule and dorsal rim of the trapezoid, rather than on the pre-existing stretched capsular and periosteal tissues (Fig. 9A and B).

If the K-wire protrudes excessively through the capsular repair, it should be trimmed so as to lie, without tension, under the skin in the antero-radial aspect of the thenar eminence. The skin is approximated with 0.7 metric (6–0 USP) no absorbable monofilament sutures, and the wrist and thumb immobilized in a plaster cast leaving the interphalangeal joint free. The cast and sutures are removed 7 to 10 days postoperatively. If the patient wishes, and just for postoperative comfort, the immobilization can be prolonged for 3 weeks. The K-wire is usually removed 5 weeks after the surgery, although a few patients, for professional or other personal reasons, had the K-wire transfixing the implant for several months without any deleterious effect on the silicone (Fig. 10A and B).

5. Conclusions

Replacement of the trapezium with a silicone implant prevents thumb ray collapse and provides recovery of painless joint mobility within a short postoperative time.

Implant subluxation can be prevented by using the smallest-sized implant, "concavization" of the trapezoid and stabilization with a circular slip of the FCR tendon which is carefully sutured to the scaphoid capsule. Transfixing the implant to the trapezoid with a Kirschner wire ensures implant stabilization during capsular healing.

Fluoroscopic examination done on patients in who had a silicone trapezium implant to replace the trapezium, demonstrated that thumb mobility was mostly taking place at the stem of the implant, same as in a flexible implant used for the MP joints. Following this observation, we allowed the patients to use the thumb early after surgery, as the body of the implant is stabilized by the Kirschner wire until capsular healing is obtained. This offers the advantage of minimizing postoperative disability, earlier return to previous occupation and faster recovery of strength and mobility.

Acknowledgements

The author thanks Profs. Gil FJ, Planell JA, Sevilla P and Proubasta I. for their analysis of a trapezium silicone implant for mechanical failure under compressive and torsion forces using a MTS Bionix 858 testing device and TestStar II® software (Center of Investigation on Biomedical Engineering. University of Barcelona).

References

[1] E.A. Nalebuff, Diagnosis, classification and management of rheumatoid hand deformities, Bull. Hosp. Joint Dis. 29 (1968) 119–137.

[2] A.E. Flatt, The thumb, in: A.E. Flatt (Ed.), The Care of the Arthritic Hand, Quality Medical Publishing, Inc, St. Louis, 1995, pp. 320–342.

[3] A.E. Flatt, The thumb, in: A.E. Flatt (Ed.), The Care of the Arthritic Hand, Quality Medical Publishing, Inc, St. Louis, 1995, p. 325.

[4] V.D. Pellegrini, R.I. Burton, Surgical management of basal joint arthritis of the thumb: Part II. Ligament reconstruction with tendon interposition arthroplasty, J. Hand Surg. 11A (1986) 324–332.

[5] A.B. Stein, A.L. Terrono, The rheumatoid thumb, Hand Clin. 12 (1996) 541–550.

[6] A.B. Swanson, Disabling arthritis at the base of the thumb. Treatment by resection of the trapezium and flexible (silicone) implant arthroplasty, J. Bone Jt. Surg. 54A (1972) 456–471.

[7] A. Lluch, Silicone spacers, in: B.R. Simmen, Y. Allieu, A. Lluch, J.K. Stanley (Eds.), Hand Arthroplasties, Marin Dunitz, London, 2000, pp. 233–242.

[8] G.D. Lister, et al., Arthritis of the trapezial articulations treated by prosthetic replacement, Hand 9 (1977) 117–118.

[9] V.D. Pellegrini, R.I. Burton, Surgical management of basal joint arthritis of the thumb: Part I. Long term results of silicone implant arthroplasty, J. Hand Surg. 11A (1986) 309–323.

[10] B.W. Connolly, S. Rath, Revision procedures for complications of surgery for osteoarthritis of the carpometacarpal joint of the thumb, J. Hand Surg. 18B (1993) 533–539.

[11] J.J. Creighton, J.B. Steichen, J.W. Strickland, Long term evaluation of silastic trapezial arthroplasty in patients with osteoarthritis.

[12] K. Hirakawa, et al., Isolation and quantification of debris particles around failed silicone orthopedic implants, J. Hand Surg. 21A (1996) 819–827.

[13] D.H. De Heer, S.R. Owens, A.B. Swanson, The host response to silicone elastomer implants for small joint arthroplasty, J. Hand Surg. 20A (1995) S101–S109.

[14] C.A. Peimer, et al., Reactive synovitis after silicone arthroplasty, J. Hand Surg. 11A (1986) 624–638.

[15] A.B. Swanson, et al., Failed carpal bone implant arthroplasty: causes and treatments, J. Hand Surg. 14A (1989) 417–424.

Author index

Keyword index